# M_CONCEPT

# M_CONCEPT

## by Laura San Martín

The model that has r**EVOLUTION**ized the management of dental practices through excellence and innovation

**M_Concept. The revolutionary dental management model**
**Laura San Martin**


ISBN: 978-1-957260-15-0
eISBN: 978-1-957260-16-7

Cover, Layout and Copyediting: Grupo Asís Biomedia S.L., Zaragoza, Spain
Project Manager: Carlos Garín Gómez, Grupo Asís Biomedia S.L., Zaragoza, Spain



**Edra Publishing US LLC**
3309 Northlake Boulevard, Suite 203
Palm Beach Gardens, FL, 33403
EIN: 844113980
info@edrapublishing.com
www.edrapublishing.com

edra
PUBLISHING

Printed by *"Masquelibros" S.L., Jaén (Andalusia)*, Spain, September 2022

# Author

Laura San Martín is a Doctor of Dentistry with European mention. Dr. San Martín also was honored with an Extraordinary Doctorate Award in Health Sciences. Her line of research was based on the improvement of diagnostic and therapeutic methods from the perspective of Minimally Invasive Dentistry (MID).

In the field of teaching, she was accredited as a full professor by the National Quality Assessment and Accreditation Agency (Agencia Nacional de Evaluación de la Calidad y Acreditación, ANECA), has been responsible for undergraduate courses and was coordinator and director of postgraduate courses. She has collaborated with national institutions and universities —University of Seville (US), King Juan Carlos University (Universidad Rey Juan Carlos, URJC), San Antonio de Murcia Catholic University (Universidad Católica San Antonio de Murcia, UCAM) or Miguel de Cervantes European University (Universidad Europea Miguel de Cervantes, UEMC)— and internationally —Harvard School of Dental Medicine (HSDM), The Forsyth Institute, World Health Organization (WHO), World Federation of Public Health Associations (WFPHA), the Council of European Chief Dental Officers (CECDO), Health and Social Care Board and Queen's University, among others—.

Her research profile has allowed her to be director of research groups in dentistry, a member of ethics committees, article reviewer for impact factor journals, a doctoral thesis and a final degree project (FDP) examiner.

She has authored numerous scientific articles, co-authored chapters and authored four books. In recent years she has been an international speaker, with more than fifty contributions to scientific congresses.

Her business profile includes the founding of SOHO dental®, SOHO Academy®, MBA dental®, Dental LifeStyle® and BŌ & BÚ. She is also cofounder of Dental Genetics®, a company specialized in genetic analysis for dental practices.

Her excellent and innovative professional career has been recognized, and she has received awards in academia, research and business.

She and her team have designed M_CONCEPT, a unique management model based on differentiation through excellence and innovation. This model has been developed by MBA dental®, the first MBA (*Master in Business Administration*) geared towards dentists in Europe and Latin America, based on this model.

# Foreword by Brian J. Swann

WATCH

Video
Brian J. Swann

There are several types of people on our planet—those who have ideas, those who talk, those who plan, and those who "do." Several years ago, I was invited by the University of Sevilla to a national meeting in Madrid as a faculty member representing the Harvard School of Dental Medicine's collaboration on preventive dentistry. During that visit, I met Dr. Laura San Martin. It became apparent to me that Dr. San Martin was a "doer." She spoke of her varied interests and her aspiration to achieve the highest levels of education and professionalism. I learned that this charismatic young doctor was passionate and fearless, that she was driven to not only accomplish her goals but also to bring her dreams to fruition. Dr. San Martin was one of the youngest students in Spain to acquire a Ph.D. and professorship in addition to obtaining her dental degree. Through determination, credibility, and networking, she would fulfill the dream of studying at the Harvard School of Dental Medicine and subsequently conduct research at the Forsyth Institute.

Upon returning to Boston, I seeked for the dean of the Harvard School of Dental Medicine. In sharing the excitement of my own professional experience in Madrid with the dean, I also discussed this young doctor I had met, who shared her enthusiasm for oral healthcare and aspired to study at Harvard. I indicated that she was among a small number of young professors with dual degrees and that she possessed a strong desire to raise the bar in her educational experiences. Having reviewed her curriculum vitae, the dean agreed that Dr. San Martin would be an asset to our university and that she should come. Within a few weeks, Dr. San Martin was a visiting lecturer at the Harvard School of Dental Medicine in the Department of Oral Health Policy and Epidemiology. Through a collaboration with the Forsyth Institute, she worked diligently over the following months and developed significant research. She would eventually publish with such collaborators as Drs. R. Niederman and T. Valente through the Centre of Evidence-Based Dentistry on the development of using social network analysis to optimize oral health prevention programs that impact early childhood oral disease, and with Dr. M. Tavares on the relationship between systemic disease and oral health. Shortly thereafter, she gained membership to the World Federation of Public Health Associations. She hosted and mentored a Harvard dental student for a research externship working on oral disease among children. Today that student is a practicing pediatric oral physician on a global level. Dr. San Martin made lasting friendships as she matured in experience and power.

During visits to a favorite SOHO café in New York City, Dr. San Martin began developing a unique and innovative concept for how she envisioned a dental care delivery system. At the core would be an evidence-based, patient-centered care model. On the business side, she incorporated customer-oriented sales with production and social network analysis methods. This led to the creation of the SOHO dental practice where she now provides comprehensive oral healthcare.

Dr. San Martin's book, *M-Concept*, is an example of her ability to bring vision to reality. Her energy and excitement for the profession, her concern for the many people who do not have access to quality oral healthcare, her willingness to share and to traverse uncharted territory have culminated in this insightful and inspiring book. It is an expression of her passion for excellence, of her care for her clients and the patients they serve. She provides cutting-edge tools for marketing that are simple and attainable. This book presents vital methods that produce success through a business model that helps ensure a balanced lifestyle.

It is my hope that Dr. San Martin will keep the good news coming, that she will continue to do the work that provides us with researched data to inform best practices and minimally invasive procedures for patients. In doing so, she will continue to support all of us as healthcare providers, our staff, and above all, the patients. Dr. San Martin is raising the standard of excellence. I trust that she will continue this trajectory. Sail onward, Dr. Laura San Martin!

*Brian J. Swann, DDS, MPH*
*Assistant Professor, Harvard School of Dental Medicine Consultant,*
*Cambridge Health Alliance*
*Joseph L. Henry Fellow*

# Foreword by Iván Malagón

WATCH

Video
Iván Malagón

It's all about saving time. And time is the ultimate wealth...

Let me explain: if someone told you to put 50 euros in a little box, an exorbitant price for a book, and two years later, when you opened that little box, you didn't have 50 euros, but 150,000 euros, everyone would put the money in, right? Well, that's what will happen if you read M_CONCEPT. Period.

Nowadays, it is difficult to find things that bring new concepts or fresh ideas, people who improve you just by existing..., and people who are on Earth to bring value in a completely altruistic way. Well, if you have a coffee with Laura San Martín that will happen to you and reading this book is like having coffee with Laura for a week, with the insomnia that it would cause you... And the fact is that writing a book telling your most intimate secrets, your knowledge from many years, everything that your mentors and the special people you have met have passed on to you, having a very awake mind, is one of the greatest proofs of generosity that exist.

The world needs more people like this. At 43 years old, I have had the opportunity to meet people of all colors: people who pass through your life without pain or glory, and who go just as they come; people who contribute to you, while making it pleasant, which is no small thing; and people you want to be close to because they add to you, because the mere fact of their existence makes you better. One of the classic ways to build success in the business world is to take as a model those people who are a reference for you, who have already achieved before you what could become your ideal of success or your goal. We all know how hard it is to find people like that: good, intelligent people. Laura is a good, intelligent person.

Getting into the subject, you probably still don't know that you need this book you are holding in your hands. You probably think that you already know everything because you are an experienced dentist or even think that the contents of this publication will not be of any use to you, because you are not a dentist... Nothing could be further from the truth.

I must say that the only sentence in the entire book that I do NOT agree with Dr. San Martín about is this one: "M_CONCEPT arises from the need for dentists to acquire specific knowledge in management and to establish an efficient and a model easy to be implemented". It is not that I disagree with what this sentence means or the way it is expressed, or even because I believe that acquiring specific knowledge in management or in establishing an efficient and easily implementable model is not really important; the reason I disagree with the author of this book is because, in my opinion, based on my experience of more than 20 years dealing with fellow dentists, the vast majority of dentists do not have that need, because they think that receiving technical knowledge and managing it in practice is enough to be successful. To have a need for something is to know that that something is an essential part of your business, your training or your person, and that is very rare in the dental profession. We may wonder why, if dentists need an office to practice their profession —i.e. a company— they do not pay at least the same level of attention to their technical training as a businessperson as they do to their technical training as a dentist, and I think it is mainly because, historically, until 30 years ago, whoever became a dentist got rich within a few years... But the refrain of La Cabra Mecánica [The Mechanical Goat] did so much damage with chorus: "You, who are so beautiful and so smart, you, who deserves a prince or a dentist!" And it didn't matter if you were a good dentist, if you were friendly or not, if you took into account important details such as making people feel good when they passed through your hands, if you were clean and took care of your image, you didn't even have to worry about whether someone was going to come through the door of your practice, because that happened almost by default. There were so few dentists that there was a huge piece of the pie for each of them, and, of course, when all is said and done, you didn't need to try hard.

Nowadays, you not only need to be a good dentist, trained at the best universities, up-to-date with the latest technologies, monitor social networks and brand positioning, worry about offering your patients increasingly better, more conservative and less invasive solutions, achieve the results your patients are looking for, and even exceed their expectations. The success of a dental practice today begins long before a patient sits in the dental chair and will depend on many aspects that have little to do with providing good treatment, which we expect to happen, of course.

That is where M_CONCEPT will be very useful for you, since it will give you a broad vision of everything you need to know to start a business without leaving any loose ends, so that you do not have to fail in things that others have already failed in and that they do not teach you at the university, to make your dental practice, your company, a profitable endeavor. Thanks to this, success will not depend on your intuition or the enthusiasm you put into your project yourself, neither your father's advice. You have the guide to success in your hands, a guide that will allow you to build things consistently.

You will hear a thousand times from your friends or people you come across: "I should have been a dentist," insinuating that being a dentist would have been a better life for them, as if all dentists were doing well..., well, nothing could be further from the truth. Unfortunately, it is because of this unfortunate belief that many people study dentistry today —i.e., to become rich overnight—. Thousands of graduates come into the market every year for whom there are no longer even the crumbs of a small piece of the old cake, and who are forced to "prostitute" themselves as *low-cost* dentists, working exploited by volume and with a shameful economic recognition that clashes head-on with the possibility of providing good treatment. If you didn't know this, if you thought this was going to be "first time's the charm," you were very wrong..., but you are lucky (even if there is no such thing as luck) to hold this book, to which you are going to dedicate the time it deserves because, now, we have created the need for you.

By now, it should be clear to you that you have to do many things, apart from technical training as a dentist, to achieve your goals and also that the classic management models are no longer effective today, because everything changes too fast; you can't stop for a moment because, the moment you stop, you'll be overtaken. M_CONCEPT will train you to respond with agility to the situations you will face.

In my book, *Eres un crack* [You're a crack] (Alienta Ed., Planeta DeAgostini), I talk a lot about taking care of your personal brand, which I consider essential to being successful and which must be built with a strategy to define who we want to be and, what is extremely important, how to be perceived as such. In my opinion, this strategy should be based on five pillars (keep these five "P's" in your head):

1. Personality: shows who you are.
2. Product: define what you offer.
3. Public: specify who you want to target.
4. Positioning: determine how you want to be perceived.
5. Promotion: communicate your personal brand.

M_CONCEPT is the best guide I have found to set you on an effective roadmap, and you should know that this is not just a book; this is the formula for superpowers, because he who has the information has the power. But now you should ask yourself: Am I ready to initiate change? The answer is: yes. You will never find a better time for this, because you have already understood that whatever doesn't evolve dies.

However, the great thing about Laura's work is that most of the ideas she presents are useful for anyone, whether you are a dentist or a hairdresser, and just reading it can be very useful. And the fact is, no matter what you do, every word in M_CONCEPT should become your "personal Bible" starting today, if you want to improve in any professional (and personal) aspect of your life, of course.

OK, let's say you already have a dental practice that works; you may even grow every year and feel comfortable thinking you have it all together... Well, throughout my life if there is one thing I have learned: The moment you feel comfortable in any situation, you have to run away from it, because from that moment on you are vulnerable because you relax, and there is nothing worse for a predator than to relax, because there is always another predator with the same hunger as you —or even more— and turns you into a prey. You may not be restless, or have never been so, when it comes to wanting to educate yourself on ways to optimize your resources, improve your practice's performance or make yourself more efficient; I am and always have been. I have read a lot of books, watched a lot of videos and attended a lot of lectures, but I have never come across a book so complete and so interesting in my life. And to you, whether you're a dentist or not, it's going to look the same.

Let's put ourselves in a very different situation from the previous one: you don't even have a practice, you're not a dentist and you think that, since you don't own a business, this is not going to do you any good. So let me clarify: whatever you do in life, you are an entrepreneur and you have to act like one. After all, an entrepreneur is nothing more than a person who has specific objectives and decides on a specific strategy to achieve them: the entrepreneur invests capital (knowledge, time or money) and work for the purpose of offering a product (you should know that your best asset is yourself) to the market in order to obtain a profit, which does not necessarily have to be cash or valuables. In fact, from my point of view, if your main goal is to get rich, you will end up skipping many of the intermediate steps that Laura tells us about in M_CONCEPT, which are necessary to achieve it. On the other hand, if the purpose behind your daily effort is to create something that others don't need because it doesn't yet exist, but that they will eventually need, you will make much more money. Above all, do not lose focus: if you are only enthusiastic about money, your impatience and the great difficulties, doubts and crises that you will encounter during the process will make you give up prematurely.

I am tired of hearing phrases like: "The competition is so intense that we've had to lower our prices." I hear this almost every day when I ask people how their business is doing. Indeed, in developed countries everything is just a click away and, at any time and quickly, you can have at your disposal everything you need: lawyers, dentists, clothing stores or hotels.

In response to the phrase in quotation marks above, I always like to clarify that there is a lot of competition among mediocrity, among those who offer services of little value, among those who demand little of themselves because they finish their day having met the minimum requirements. The mass is unqualified because "qualification" requires a lot of effort and dedication and because it is much more comfortable to be on the couch watching garbage on a cell phone or TV than to take action with the number of ideas and advice provided by Dr. San Martín, which requires courage, perseverance and a lot of patience in order to understand that, little by little, enormous things can be built.

As soon as you start reading M_CONCEPT you will discover that you have to differentiate yourself, that you have to do what others don't do, so that the target audience you have defined chooses you. The individual who takes refuge in a "herd" society, who acts like the rest and who does not want to leave their comfort zone is really looking for the security that comes from belonging to a community, feeling part of something and giving meaning to their existence because they feels more comfortable around others who think like them. As such, they just take up space, but contribute nothing, only mass volume. In your hand, between these pages, is the perfect map to set yourself apart from the rest, to make your practice a place made in your image and likeness that makes every person who steps in and puts their oral health in your hands feel special.

Still don't realize how lucky you are? Don't you know how much time and work M_CONCEPT is saving you? The value of such a book is incalculable! There is no better investment than one that can exponentially multiply your wealth, whether personal or financial, and, as I begin this prologue, I promise you that the 50 euros you spend will multiply by hundreds of thousands.

However, effort is not pleasant; it is much more comfortable and relaxed not to lift a finger than to worry about making your dreams come true. But dreams only come true if you work your tail off to achieve them. Mr. Walt Disney said: "If you can dream it, you can do it." But good old Walt forgot to clarify that the simple fact of being able to dream it is no guarantee of anything, unless you have the necessary willpower to dedicate yourself completely to fulfilling your dream. Accordingly, and with Mr. Disney's permission, I would change his sentence to: "If you can dream it and you have the balls (or ovaries) to do the impossible to get it, you can do it." (Iván Malagón 😊).

With this simple and subtle clarification, it is clear that those who strive for excellence have little competition. But beware, because this does not mean that you should stop worrying, quite the contrary: the competition is smaller, but much tougher, among other things, because in the excellence niche one of your biggest competitors is yourself. When you have references or admire someone, you have a margin of action and you can follow a more or less defined path. However, when there is not much above you, or very little, everything becomes more complex, but at the same time more enriching; it is then that you start becoming yourself and you feel completely free to not have to look around, just straight ahead. In that moment, you can even give yourself license to be your purest self, to stop having to follow the rules that others have created and start creating them yourself. That is when the field opens up as much as you want and you take more risks in each step, and it will be from that moment on when you will feel that the accomplishment of that challenge is directly proportional to the degree of satisfaction for having achieved it.

*Iván Malagón*
*Orthodontics Expert, opinion leader and international speaker*

## ACKNOWLEDGMENTS

This book is the result of years of work. It is difficult to thank on one page all the people who are responsible for my being here today writing this book.

To my family, for their continuous support in every project I undertake. Especially to my father, for every minute he has dedicated to me, for teaching me so much and for being my constant inspiration.

To my love, for always being by my side, for taking care of me and for picking me up every time I fall.

To Brian Swann, for guiding me, for believing in me and for showing me another way to understand dentistry.

To my team, without whom none of this would be possible. Thank you for every milestone, being by your side is the best part of the finished product.

To the students at MBA dental®, for trusting us, for making us grow and for all the moments you have given us.

To all the colleagues with whom I share this profession, who make us even more passionate about dentistry.

To all the professionals who have been involved in this book, who are re-evolving dentistry with your practices.

To you, for purchasing this book.

To all of you who have been part of this project, both on the inside and the outside, THANK YOU.

## ABOUT THE BOOK

First of all, thank you for purchasing this book. We hope you really enjoy reading it as much as we have enjoyed creating it.

This publication is not intended to be a conventional book, but rather one of those readings that will lead you to reflect and make small changes; a guide that will encourage you to go beyond reading and implement actions in your dental practice through an innovative management model.

In this book we will describe step by step a model from a different perspective. We also want to show you our way of understanding dentistry, with the aim that it can be an interesting philosophy to implement in your daily life.

Over the years, colleagues and students have suggested that I write a book. At that time I was going through a *nonstop* phase of life, the kind during which you don't even have time to think about what's really important.

Sounds familiar? Surely at some point in your lifetime you have gone through this, or are currently going through something similar.

However, everything happens at the perfect time and, after years of a very intense pace of work, travel and projects, I decided to slow down. During that pause, I decided to be very careful in selecting the professional projects I would embark on, so I could dedicate more time to my personal life and so I could write this book.

What I have experienced is related to everything I am going to tell you in the following chapters. Your personal and professional lives are not independent entities, so M_CONCEPT is more than just a management model.

- To illustrate this, we will take you on a tour (*Connecting the dots*) through a series of experiences that have marked my professional career and that have led me to where I am today, writing this book.

Changing your *mindset mind or frame of mind*, having a clear vision and optimizing your most valuable resource —your time— will be the biggest takeaways you can get from this book.

For that to happen, I ask you to:

1. Read the whole book.
2. Keep the reading order.
3. Put into practice what you learn while reading.

## EXPERIENCE

Do we do something different? As I would like the reading experience to be somewhat different and more interactive, I propose the following:

- This book has interactive resources: scan the QR codes to access them.
- Listen to the playlist we have designed for **you**.

LISTEN

Playlist for M_CONCEPT

- Find your learning environment: choose the right time and place and combine them with what you enjoy (e.g. coffee).

Identifying when and with what stimuli you are most efficient will help you in the learning process, make it more enjoyable and therefore produce a greater impact.

Spend a few minutes a day, even if it's only five, but practice consistent reading. Propose a number of pages until you reach the end. It is very likely that you will read or consult this book on more than one occasion. If all this happens, when you reach chapter VI you will return to chapter I.

This book also aims to connect with professionals like you, people with intellectual curiosity and motivation, and to improve in everything you do.

As you know, we are in the digital age. For this reason, we have created a space where you can tell us in real time about your experience and share it with other professionals.

I must confess that my "yankee experience" has left its mark and in this book you will find two aspects that prove it that prove it, such as the use of abbreviations and acronyms.

The first point is due to the fact that my training and apprenticeship in *management* has been mainly in English and, with regards to the second, we have established acronyms because they are easier to assimilate and remember.

## INTRODUCTION TO M_CONCEPT

M_CONCEPT arises from the need for dentists to acquire specific knowledge in management and to establish an efficient and an easy model to implement. These aspects are essential to achieve an excellent practice and guarantee the viability of our dental practice.

This model has been developed thanks to the collaboration of a team of experts who have supported me for years and it has been improved with each version.

M_CONCEPT has been implemented in hundreds of practices, which have provided us with feedback regarding the results and improvements obtained, which has proved to be of great value to the evolution of this model.

Our goal is to enable more and more practices to develop efficient management and improve their performance through progressive implementation.

Do you know the story of Dick Fosbury? He was the athlete who revolutionized the technique of the high jump and who created the so-called *Fosbury flop*. This athlete was not the most powerful or the fastest or the tallest. He was unsatisfied with traditional techniques, so he began experimenting with a new style, with which he achieved an Olympic record and with which he changed the established rules of a discipline.

M_CONCEPT was born out of dissatisfaction with the lack of knowledge, tools and management models that allow a dentist to achieve an excellent practice.

Before delving into M_CONCEPT, there are three aspects we should focus on:

### 1 Understanding the dental care process (DCP)

The success of today's dental practice is not based solely on the excellent technical skills of the dentist.

From this premise, broaden your view:
"Think outside the dental chair."

Throughout the chapters, you will learn about the key aspects that will determine the success of your dental practice, as valued by your patients and staff.

The excellent performance of a treatment is part of the so-called *guaranteed elements*, i.e., those that refer to aspects that patients "take for granted."

In M_CONCEPT we are going to focus on distinctive elements, i.e., those that will differentiate you from your competition and allow you to expand the concept of excellence beyond the dental chair.

The provision of services also has intangible aspects, so the measurement of their experience (perceptions) is an essential factor.

For this reason, we will focus on all the non-technical aspects that you probably haven't stopped to think about and that you need to work on in order for your dental practice to achieve excellence.

Another very important aspect is that the DCP does not start when the patient sits in our chair, not even when the patient enters our practice.

Therefore, in M_CONCEPT we will work on the three phases of the care process: pre-during-post (PDP).

## 2 Efficient management

Your dental practice is a company. This concept, which seems basic, deserves a brief reflection for most dentists.

Our clinical decisions are usually based on extensive training and a high degree of scientific evidence, while business decisions are based on intuition and advice with little knowledge of the subject matter.

But let's start at the beginning: What is a company?

Josh Kaufman defines it in a way which I find very interesting:

*"A successful business (1) creates or offers something of value that others (2) need or want (3) at a price at which they are willing to pay, so that (4) it satisfies their needs and expectations, (5) which generates sufficient revenue, so that its owners find it profitable to continue operating."*

This brief definition functionally sums up what a company is and, —as you know—, also entails a commitment related to your dedication, your enthusiasm and your investment, in economic terms, as well as in terms of time and effort.

Our profession gives meaning to our lives.

Does it seem important enough?

It is essential for you to dedicate time to learning business aspects that will allow you to properly manage your dental practice and ensure its viability in the medium and long term.

Around 80% of companies fail in their first year. That is a very high percentage, especially knowing that a large number of the professionals behind them are good technicians, who did not know how to manage their companies correctly.

However, it is not enough just to get occasional training; from now on you must be up to date and renew your knowledge, so that it can be adapted to the context of each moment.

Traditional management models are no longer effective, as we are currently facing a dynamic environment full of uncertainty (VUCA*), to which we must respond with agility, flexibility and speed.

J. Paul Getty said:

*"To succeed in business, to get to the top, an individual must know everything that can be known about that business."*

Our proposal is to offer differentiated knowledge with a broad vision and comprehensive management. That is why we will approach a 360° model, based on six modules plus implementation: strategy, differentiation, analysis, core, innovation and excellence.

This model has a method and tools (M tools) that will allow you to apply the basis for the theoretical content.

The results of the implementation will be measured internally (KPIs and team satisfaction) and externally (patient satisfaction). This constitutes the Golden Triangle.

## 3 Optimization and focus on professional excellence

Our time is limited and, therefore, is the most precious asset we have to produce our activity. Therefore, we must optimize it. You can learn through a long process of mistakes, but this will lead to frustration and a loss of resources.

Our goal is to accelerate the learning process and help you avoid mistakes by modeling, i.e., to reproduce what has already been done by people/companies that have achieved excellence.

Unlike products, providing services depends on an investment of time and energy by a professional and their team; therefore, they are finite. This is something we are going to reflect on, since, although in most cases we cannot count on a scalable business model, we can increase performance, automate the DCP and improve processes.

To start on the road to excellence, we must be clear about two premises: the first is to work on a model of continuous improvement and the second is to focus our practice on the patient (patient centric).

Our efforts must be oriented towards the satisfaction of our patients through an excellent practice, thereby obtaining an economic benefit.

Therefore, revenue is the result, not the objective. This change of focus is the starting point.

Most dental practices play the minimum game, i.e., they offer the minimum possible in order to compete. All patients take it for granted that we will solve their dental problems, but that is not an exceptional value, it is what they expect; that is why, in this model, we are going to focus on providing something more.

The next level should be based on performing a correct practice (doing things well). We propose that you take a leap forward towards professional excellence, i.e.**exceed** the **expectations** of your **patients**, which will be the element that will make the difference in your dental practice.

Most practices can access these three levels, but due to lack of knowledge, organization or communication, they do not focus their practice correctly.

When I ask my students at MBA dental® what is their main objective for being in the master's program, a large majority of them answered: "To increase my practice's profits." This is a flawed focus. We will modify this as we progress through the program, and I hope it will also happen as you read this book.

** VUCA is an acronym for volatile, uncertainty, complex and ambiguous.*

Remember that the ability for a work team to achieve excellence lies in its leader, i.e. in you! Therefore, it is important for you to acquire specific knowledge in this area and transversal skills —beyond the dental chair— that will help you achieve the professional success associated with your talent and good clinical practice.

## FEEDBACK ABOUT MANAGEMENT

#iamabusinessperson

Being a good manager will help you become a better dentist. The reason for the existence of any dental practice is to provide excellent service to its patients. Optimal management will connect you to that goal. I understood this aspect years ago and have since approached my clinical practice differently.

Usually, dentists do not identify with "being entrepreneurs," and due to a lack of knowledge, we even have a negative perception of this term. I myself, at another point in my career, despite being the leader of more than one practice, had no specific business training and rejected the term *entrepreneur*, instead preferring the term dentist.

Today's concept is holistic: being a good dentist means being a good entrepreneur, in a bidirectional way.

On some occasions, for many dentists, the entrepreneurial initiative involved in a dental practice is passive (they consider it to be their only professional outlet, they are continuing a family project...), so they identify themselves as forced entrepreneurs. In other situations, it is an intuitive process (with no knowledge or specific training) full of trial and error.

The *status quo* we are going to show you is that of a successful entrepreneur, whose mission is to improve peoples' lives through their talent, practiced with ethical criteria, commitment and responsibility.

When you finish this book, I hope that your vision will change and you will realize that a good entrepreneur, who strives for excellence, is trained, is involved, cares about their team, is committed to continuous improvement and offers the highest level of care to their patients is a better dentist.

For this, there is a very effective exercise which is to "open our mind" and "depart our wonderful tooth world". This is the environment where we are at ease, because it represents our passion, and what we do best. This, in the business world, is called

"Getting out of our comfort zone."

When we leave our practice and have a different perspective, we start to learn from everything that happens outside those four walls: we observe what other companies are doing, get inspired by any experience, write down ideas during our travels...

Probably the most valuable thing you will gain by finishing this book is to broaden your perspective. It took me several experiences to get here and, although I wouldn't change any of them, I now know that there is a more direct path.

I'm sure you've heard on more than one occasion Steve Jobs' famous theory, which he shared in his commencement speech to Stanford University students, entitled *the dots*.

I often think of it, especially when I remember situations that have marked my trajectory, seemingly unconnected, but that have led me to the point where I am today.

In my American experience I wanted to grow personally and professionally, beyond dentistry, to which I devoted 100% of my time, energy and interest.

Therefore, during that period, I decided to invest part of my limited free time in expanding my knowledge in those unexplored areas that were not directly related to the dental sector.

That's when I started enrolling in courses and seminars, attending talks… At that time, I was living between Boston and New York, which are two cities with a lot of activity, where you have the opportunity to meet people from all over the world with incredible projects and around whom it was very easy to get inspired.

I could tell you many anecdotes about situations in which my restlessness led me and in which I really thought: *What am I doing here? Or, even better: Why am I not in my office, where I like to be, where I feel safe and where I enjoy myself?!*

When you find yourself surrounded by Harvard Business School (HBS) gurus, it's easy to feel out of your comfort zone. If we add to that a mentor with very effective methods who will get the best out of you, but with a tough process…, the desire to return to the office increases!

During those months, the phrase that I heard most often in videoconferences with my family and friends was: *But why are you doing this?* At that time, it was difficult to see the point of a dentist attending courses in marketing, programming and theater, or volunteer work in a cheese factory (yes, you read it right!). Because marketing was for those working in marketing departments; programming, for computer scientists; theater, for actors; and the cheese factory, for its workers.

Now I can say, connecting these experiences, that each and every one of them provided me with invaluable learning and has had a great impact on my professional and personal career.

I feel very fortunate to have had the opportunity to meet great professionals who have "forced" me out of my comfort zone and who have shown me that another perspective was possible.

However, on this road to excellence, not everything is success, and these people also taught me how to fail. It is possibly one of the most important lessons I have learned in recent years.

One of my biggest fears as an entrepreneur was failure; I understood it as a place that, if you get there, shows a lack of talent, a point where your idea-project, to which you have dedicated so much time and enthusiasm, collapses. Now I understand failures as the best source of learning and growth, and as an opportunity to continue with more knowledge.

With this book I hope to be able to pass on to you the importance of management in our profession. I also hope that my experience can serve you without you having to get stressed out among a bunch of CEOs of large multinational companies! (just kidding: experience more than recommended.) If I succeed, you won't be able to imagine dentistry without management.

In the following chapters we will share our vision with you and show you everything that management can bring to your entrepreneurial process; a process that, without knowing it, you started years ago, even before you had your practice.

In this book we won't focus on me, but on you, on your team, on your project, on your dental practice. If you are reading this book it is because you have that entrepreneurial restlessness or because you are a professional with a desire to improve, and that is already the first characteristic that differentiates you from your competition.

In this book we will describe, through the M_CONCEPT model, a work philosophy with a specific method. We are going to provide you with the knowledge and some business management tools to put you at the forefront of the dental industry if you apply them effectively.

To this end, we will share with you specific aspects that will allow you to develop the necessary skills to properly "pilot" your dental practice and achieve sustained success, even in an environment essentially characterized by great dynamism, high competition and uncertainty.

## GUIDELINES

This is not just a book; it is the beginning of change.

This book will broaden your knowledge in management, but, in addition, I propose that reading this will help you to reflect, analyze and execute it.

For that, two factors must occur:

- Change your *mindset*: with this book I hope to offer you a content providing you with another perspective on how to understand dentistry.

*"Reading is thinking with someone else's brain instead of one's own."*
*Arthur Schopenhauer*

- Move to action: it is important that, as you progress through the M_CONCEPT model, you implement the *tips* and make use of the tools (Mc_tools) that we offer you.

*"Learning is not memorizing, it is learning by doing."*
*Howard Gardner*

A book can change the way we think, feel and act. Reading activates certain areas of the brain involved in learning and decision-making. The activation that occurs in certain regions of the brain when reading is similar to that which occurs when events happen in reality.

In other words: your mind becomes suggestible, perceives and reproduces an action even before it happens.

We hope to inspire you with this book, beyond its pages.

**Less is more: three ideas**

Communication experts say that humans are capable of effectively retaining three ideas; therefore, in each chapter I will summarize the three key concepts that you should not forget after each reading.

In this book you will notice that we will spend little time on the external context (saturation, competition, franchises...) in order to focus on you and your practice.

Given the same environment, the way you manage it will determine the results.

Therefore, although our approach will be eminently internal, the external context will help us detect opportunities, minimize risks and identify trends. This analysis requires an important reflection that we are sometimes unwilling to undertake as entrepreneurs.

To do so, I ask only one thing of you: You have to get through the first chapter! Because this is the step you probably skipped in your entrepreneurial project.

During this entrepreneurial training, will be your first day's stiffness! But, if you overcome it, the flow will begin, in which you will enjoy every step leading you to success.

Jordan Ellenberg is a mathematician at the University of Wisconsin who analyzed the number of readers who stop reading a *best seller* before reaching the last page. During this study, he determined that those with scientific or economic themes are the most frequently abandoned. And they were best sellers! However, 70% of people who get past page 50 finish the book.

We value your time enormously, so we intend to make this an enjoyable and useful read. To this end, we have included attractive elements that will motivate you to finish this book, because we really think it will be important for you to get to the end.

Through Mc_experience you will have access to:

- Mc_videos: short videos of people who will enrich your reading.
- Mc_tools: templates with examples and practical implementation.
- Mc_senses: audiovisual elements that will make your reading more enjoyable.
- Mc_route & goal: a personal path to a real goal (*dots & connecting the dots*).

You will be able to access these elements via QR codes that you will find in each section and that you must scan using your cell phone camera.

In order to give you a very practical and real management perspective, we have included the section *Connecting the dots*. At the beginning of each chapter you will be able to read a story (*dot*) which, connected to the rest, gives meaning to the final result. As you progress through the reading, you will be closer to understanding the objective. Thus, I hope to make sure you make it to the end, without skipping any chapters!

Before we begin, I'd like you to watch the speech Steve Jobs gave at Stanford University, in which he talks about the theory of *Connecting the dots* and how it marked his career.

WATCH

Video
Steve Jobs:
*Connecting the dots*

Do you remember when we were in school, learning to draw, we used to connect dots and a picture would appear at the end? You could only see the result if you linked them all in order. This will be similar.

Shall we begin?

# Content

# STRATEGY

## What you should know before starting

Listen to *Bloodflow*,
by Grandbrothers

Reading time:
48 minutes

# M

the

Reading time: 6 min

# Strategy is a pattern in a stream of decisions*

*"Why have you ruled out studying medicine? It's the career you've wanted since you were a child and you obtained the entry grade."*

*My father has always been my model and his passion for medicine has been passed on to my sister and myself since we were little.*

*He is one of those doctors with a vocation, who cares for his patients and is concerned about them inside and outside the office. He is now retired, but continues to read scientific articles and enjoy our clinical cases.*

*"Dad, I'd like to be my own boss.*

*Today I went to the dental practice you recommended to see the surgery and I thought I might study dentistry."*

*I have always liked surgery, so, a few months before finishing high school, I visited several operating rooms until I ended up at a dental practice. The day I visited the office implant surgery had been scheduled. It was the first time I had attended a procedure of this nature*

*For an hour, my attention was divided between the surgery and the way a synchronized team performed each step until the treatment was completed.*

*After the surgery, I had the opportunity to remain at the clinic. It was then when I decided I wanted to be a dentist.*

*Henry Mintzberg* stated that strategy is not the consequence of planning: on the contrary, it is the starting point.*

*"A company without a strategy is willing to try anything."*
*Michael Porter*

The management of dental practices has attracted growing interest in recent years, especially those professionals who have realized the importance of adequately optimizing all their resources and who are committed to continuous improvement, focusing on a model of professional excellence.

The viability of a dental practice can only be achieved by applying the right mechanisms for correct and efficient business management.

Management remains unfinished business for most dentists. This is due to several factors, the most important of which include the low teaching load in academic programs and the prioritization, interest or focus of dentists on eminently technical or clinical learning.

This gap, or lack of knowledge, has led to the instability of many dental practices, and has directly affected them in terms of profitability and optimization.

I must admit that I was one of those dentists with little interest in management. When I started training in this area, it not only changed the way I understood dentistry, but also had a great impact on the performance and quality of my professional practice.

From our perspective, management is a must, an obligation we dentists have to our patients, our dental practice and our profession.

I hope that reading this book will be the beginning of your interest in this subject, which is so exciting and important for a dentist.

As you know, our environment is highly competitive and characterized by great dynamism, which makes it essential for a dentist and their team to be adequately prepared and adapted.

To start building a solid foundation, the first step is to focus on the strategy. Most dental practices do not have a defined strategy and, therefore, no direction to guide them towards their objectives.

Mentioning this term sounds like "big business" to most dentists; they consider strategic processes to be the domain of another type of business.

That is the first mistake: all companies must have a strategy. From this moment on, you should know that part of your dedication, if you really want to achieve success, will be based on defining it, reviewing it and sitting down at least once a week to follow up on it.

If you do it the right way, your office time will be more profitable than your couch time. I know what you're thinking: As a dentist, only your chair time production is more profitable. Well, I must inform you that the numbers and the results show otherwise.

Probably, even if you are not yet familiar with this concept, you have already taken some action related to it before opening your dental practice. Strategic processes must also be reviewed and developed on an ongoing basis.

In this book, you will learn how to guide your dental practice towards excellence using a strategic approach, and you will acquire simple concepts and tools that will be incredibly useful in your daily management.

1 2 3 4 5 6 7 result

# Building a solid foundation: MVV

Reading time: 8 min

*"A good strategy starts by having the right objective."*
*Michael Porter*

Let's start at the beginning: strategy.

Business strategy is the starting point of any entrepreneurial process, so if you have a dental practice, as in any business, the first thing you must define is an objective and a roadmap to achieve it.

For that, you need to have a foundation on which to begin to build and grow, which is called a *strategic plan*. In dentistry, it is not very common to find a dental practice that has defined and established this foundation prior to the start of its activity.

Subsequently, you must work on the way in which the actions will be developed or executed, having a method; i.e., designing your business tactics.

The determining factor for your dental practice to improve results, adapt to change and be properly managed depends on your vision.

Not having short-, medium- and long-term goals and not knowing where you are headed as a business will have a major impact on the viability and survival of your dental practice.

Strategy is a decision model that establishes the philosophy, actions and adequacy of resources to meet the proposed objectives and allows for the anticipation, control and forecasting of results.

In M_CONCEPT, we will rely on the OKR (Objectives and Key Results) system, which is a method that will allow you to achieve strategic goals efficiently.

## MISSION, VISION AND VALUES

The first step in establishing a strategy is to define the mission, vision and values (MVV) of your clinic, through an explicit statement shared with both your patients and your staff.

Defining the MVV in writing will allow you to better orient your strategy, establish priorities and mark your actions.

The **mission** defines the purpose, the raison d'être; i.e., your work or activity in the market. It should be focused on the target audience and on the uniqueness, particularity or differential factor through which the activity is developed.

I know what you're thinking: As a dentist, only your chair time production is more profitable. Some questions that can help you define your clinic's mission are: *what do you do?, what does your service bring to the market?, who is your goal or audience?, what is your geographic scope of action?, what is your competitive advantage?, what differentiates you from your competitors?*

For example, the mission described by Google is to organize information in the world to make it useful and accessible.

The **vision** defines the goals you intend to achieve, where you are heading and, therefore, your aspirations.

Every clinic has a beginning, but aims to evolve. The vision must be inspiring, attractive and easily remembered. However, this goal must also be realistic and achievable, since the vision proposal is motivational in nature.

*"One can only progress when they think big, we can only move forward when we look further on."*

*José Ortega y Gasset*

Returning to the previous example, Google's vision is to position itself as the most important search engine in the world.

As you can see, the mission places you in the present and the vision in the future. That is, who you are now and who you want to become.

To establish your clinic's vision, it will help to answer the following questions: *What do you want to achieve, where do you see your clinic in a few years, what will your dental practice become in the future, where do you want to be in the future, how much will you expand your area of operation?*

And lastly, **values**, are ethical principles on which the culture of your clinic is based and which allow you to create your own behavioral guidelines.

Values are the personality of our clinic.

You should try to make those values attractive and differentiating and, of course, align them with your own values, what you believe in. It is not a good idea to formulate more than five or six values.

Questions such as: *what do we believe in? or, what are we like?* will help you define your corporate values.

Some of the values most commonly used by companies are commitment, quality, passion, proximity... These should also be aligned with your team and your patients.

Google's values are speed, accuracy, good customer service, innovation and ease of use.

The **mission**, **vision** and **values** must be consistent with each other. It is also important that they be written down and made public, for example, on your clinic's website.

I know what you're thinking: As a dentist, only your chair time production is more profitable.

WATCH

Video Dr. Lewischen: *The importance of having a vision*

Top management gurus define the MVV as corporate DNA or identity, which gives coherence, authenticity and originality or differentiation to your company.

Defining what type of clinic we are will be the basis for determining the rest of the actions we will carry out.

These terms can be written on a sheet of paper, so we suggest that you write them on the template provided and start writing them today, if you have not already done so. If you have already defined them, you can review and redefine them if you consider it appropriate.

DOWNLOAD

Template 1: *MVV*

It usually takes the form of a statement of purpose, which should be easy to remember, forceful and, therefore, relatively brief.

In short, you must have a strategic vision that guides the activity to be developed in your dental practice.

If you think of a brand that you consume frequently, even if there are cheaper options —i.e. a brand motivating your loyalty— you will probably find it is a company committed to its MVV, where there is a connection between product/service, employees and customers.

You are and will be a promoter of the forementioned brand, therefore, you will recommend it to other people.

That will be your ultimate goal, for your potential patients to know about your work and for current patients to recommend you, since it is the best indication of having successfully completed all phases of the care process, achieving their satisfaction and loyalty.

1 2 3 4 5 6 7 result

# Your dental practice´s strategic diagnosis

Reading time: 10 min

In order to propose a valid strategy, you must have a global and integral vision of your dental practice, both externally and internally.

Your dental practice´s strategic diagnosis.

Your dental practice´s strategic diagnosis. Ideally, you should be able to anticipate or adapt quickly to future changes affecting your clinic.

This analysis will allow you to work on a new strategic paradigm and to refocus or realign resources through rapid responses to all these changes.

In this changing environment, new management approaches and flexible methods are emerging that allow you to adapt to new scenarios. (*Lean*, Agile/Scrum methodology, *Kanban* methodology).

Based on these methodologies, we have adapted our management model and incorporated those tools that are useful to a dental practice.

Most innovative methods arise in the industrial field, so their incorporation into the service sector and, specifically, into dentistry have required extensive adaptation, which we have embodied in M_CONCEPT.

## EXTERNAL AND INTERNAL ANALYSIS OF YOUR DENTAL PRACTICE

Dentists usually start a business project without carrying out a prior market study, so our consulting actions include factors that we are not going to change (for example: the location of the clinic).

If this is your case, don't worry, there is still time to adapt and boost your dental practice, as long as your vision is broad and flexible, and your actions are effective.

Ideally, you should acquire this type of knowledge prior to the entrepreneurial process and develop an initial analysis to help you estimate the probability of success.

The variables we will analyze include those that will create opportunities and those that will constitute threats.

In our model, we will focus mainly on an internal approach and on factors on which you can act, but we will not ignore external analysis, which will be fundamental.

This approach is based on our way of understanding and dealing with management and market positioning (which we will explain in each chapter).

In the external analysis, i.e., the evaluation of the environment (macro and micro environment), we will identify the main factors influencing the development or performance of your dental practice.

The macro-environment or generic environment factors are those that affect all sectors of the economy, which cannot be changed and which cannot be influenced, but which must be known (economic, technological, political, socio-cultural factors, etc.).

The factors related to the micro-environment or specific environment affect only companies in a given sector and can be controlled to a certain extent (competitors, customers, suppliers, etc.).

## MACRO-ENVIRONMENT ANALYSIS

A thorough knowledge of the environment around your clinic will help you be more competitive. There are different tools that can help you perform this analysis.

**PEST Analysis:** comprised of political, economic, social and technological factors.

DOWNLOAD

Template 2: *PEST*

**PESTEL Analysis:** in addition to the above analysis, some authors add two more dimensions: the ecological and the legal.

**SWOT Matrix:** is a simple, effective and visual method that will help you make a strategic diagnosis of your clinic and make future decisions.

The information obtained shows the state of the clinic, in terms of itself and the environment in which it develops or wishes to develop.

The name of this method corresponds to the initials: (S) strengths, (W) weaknesses, (O) opportunities and (T) threats.

In terms of internal analysis, strengths can represent competitive advantages, while weaknesses are aspects that limit or reduce the capacity for the effective development of the clinic's strategy.

Threats and opportunities are aspects of external analysis that do not depend directly on the clinic, but do affect it. Therefore, threats and opportunities must be identified and actions must be taken to act on the former and take advantage of the latter.

> This strategy is defined to enhance strengths, overcome weaknesses, control threats and benefit from opportunities.

DOWNLOAD

Template 3.1: *SWOT*

Based on the results obtained in the SWOT matrix, different types of strategies can be drawn up: defensive, offensive, survival or reorientation.

- Defensive strategy: a situation in which the clinic prepares for potential threats, which it will counter with internal resources.
- Offensive strategy: results from the intersection of strengths and opportunities. It is a situation of growth and improved market positioning. Now is the time to leverage strengths and leadership in the sector by taking advantage of a favorable framework.
- Survival strategy: results from the intersection of weaknesses and threats. It is a situation in which a prudent attitude is adopted allowing for resource management until the changes arising are stabilized.

- Reorientation strategy: results from the intersection of weaknesses and opportunities. In this situation, the clinic must identify its disability in order to take advantage of new opportunities.

DOWNLOAD

Template 3.2: *McKinsey Matrix*

With the combination of (S) (W) (O) (T) we will mark strategic lines of action.

The **McKinsey Matrix** is a tool that helps to make investment decisions based on competitive position and market attractiveness.

**CAME Analysis:** this matrix will reflect the strategies to be followed according to the results obtained in the SWOT analysis. In other words, it complements the study by channeling its results through clear and specific lines of action.

Its initials correspond to:

- (**C**) Correct weaknesses
- (**A**) Adapt to threats
- (**M**) Maintain strengths
- (**E**) Exploit opportunities

DOWNLOAD

Template 4: *CAME Analysis*

## MICRO-ENVIRONMENT ANALYSIS

**Porter's Five Forces Analysis:** this strategic model establishes a framework for analyzing the level of competition in a sector. For Michael E. Porter, the success of a company depends on its ability to take advantage of favorable external factors (opportunities) and combat unfavorable factors (threats) better than its competitors.

Competitiveness and profitability therefore determine the structure of an industry.

DOWNLOAD

Template 5: *Porter's Forces*

This tool helps us to make decisions and allows us to determine the degree of competition in our sector (comparing competitive advantages). It also allows us to formulate, design and develop appropriate strategies to achieve success, in current and future scenario.

In the following chapters you will also see innovation assisting to transform the standards of an industrial sector.

One model that integrates, from an innovative approach, the external forces that most influence business models is the one proposed by the authors Alexander Osterwalder and Yves Pigneur.

They classify them into four areas: **market forces** (needs/demands, switching costs…), **industry forces** (competitors, substitute services…), **key trends** (social, economic, technological…) and **macroeconomic forces** (global market, economic infrastructure…).

Therefore, knowing the environment will allow you to design an adapted and competitive business model. These tools provide you with an approximation of that analysis.

For a dental practice to go from good to excellent, it needs to go further than its competition. This has to do with detecting what you do better than the rest of the clinics in a given context, so you should dedicate time to this analysis.

Reading time: 16 min

# The CANVAS model in dentistry: your Business Model in one step

## KNOWING THE PULSE OF THE MARKET

This strategy involves a permanent relationship between the dental practice and its environment. Therefore, in order to define it properly, it is essential to analyze the market situation.

Whether you have started your activity or you are going to do it, you have probably designed some action, even without knowing it, related to market research.

Surely, you have compared several options before renting or buying a facility, you have investigated the number of clinics around you, you have been interested in the socioeconomic status of the population... this is part of the initial analysis for your business model.

Market research is a systematic process of collecting and analyzing data and information about patients-customers, competitors, suppliers and the market itself in order to assess the viability of our business project.

This analysis helps you to better understand the environment in which you are going to develop your activity, allows you to improve your services and guides you to expand the growth of your dental practice.

Tools are available to assess this start-up by identifying, describing and analyzing a business opportunity. To this end, we will examine their technical, economic and financial feasibility.

Whether you are going to open a practice or you want to reactivate the one you already have, you must work on a preliminary step: the business model.

The business model (BM) is intended to describe the foundation on which the clinic will create, deliver and capture value.

Some clinics simply sell, others add value.

In the following chapters, we will explain the importance and impact of focusing your strategy on value creation.

The focus, therefore, will be on generating profits based on the value proposition. To start designing it, you need to answer the following questions:

>>>> Who? The client-patient objective.

>>>> What? The value and solutions offered by your service.

>>>> How? How you will provide the service. How you are going to make a profit and with what resources.

You have probably never explicitly asked yourself a series of key questions, based on which you must validate and design your business idea.

There are different ways to offer value to patients; among them, you can focus on elements such as: personalization, innovation, performance, design, accessibility, convenience/ease of access to the service…

With this information, all the necessary procedures and strategies are developed to turn a business opportunity into a defined business project.

The *business plan* (BP) compiles the strategies to be followed to execute the business model. This involves the service proposals, marketing plans and financial operations as well as market research or positioning analysis, among others.

Just as the comprehensive diagnosis of a patient is the first step to ensure the success of a treatment, the BP is the best tool to achieve proper direction and decision-making on an objective and analytical basis, not just based on intuition, ideas or beliefs.

Therefore, in this section, we will talk about the business model (BM) and the business plan (BP). The BM is the first step to validate your idea and should be done first.

**The business model describes how your clinic will create value for patients, while earning a profit.**

The BP is the document that describes the objectives for the venture and is comprised of:

1. The business model.
2. Economic/financial viability.
3. The future projection for the third party assessment of the clinic.

**The business plan is the roadmap that marks the daily planning for your dental practice.**

The business plan will be made when you are already in operation. This document is dynamic, i.e. it should be reviewed periodically and updated as necessary.

As an exercise, we propose you to design your BM through the Canvas model. (*Business Canvas Model*), which will allow you to see its nine elements on a single sheet of paper.

The authors of this model, Alexander Osterwalder and Yves Pigneur, have created a tool that makes it easy to describe, evaluate and modify a BM.

This tool is included in his book *Business Model Generation* which we recommend if you would like more information on this subject.

It is a useful exercise that will help you position your dental practice in a competitive landscape, whether you are a new opening or an active practice that wants to innovate.

Each section of the *canvas* reflects the structure that is part of a company's revenue-producing structure. These nine modules cover the four main areas of any business, including those of a dental practice: customer-patients, supply, infrastructure and economic viability.

It is a comprehensive and visual tool that will allow you to understand and make decisions in a very simple way.

These four areas establish four basic questions that a dental practice must ask itself:

1. What are you offering? It is the center of the model, the **value proposition** of the clinic.
2. Who are you serving? These are the different **patient segments** for whom you prepare the value proposition.
3. How are you going to serve them? You must define three sections: **key activities, key resources and key partners.**
4. What will the cost be? Here you will analyze the **cost structure and sources of income** of the clinic.

The starting point of the Canvas model is the value proposition, which is what differentiates you from the market, so it is at the center of the canvas.

This value proposition is what you deliver to your patients, with whom you will have to establish a series of relationships through certain channels (for example, the Internet) or, in your case, through the dental practice itself.

Internally, there are the key activities and resources, i.e., what you must do to be able to offer the service and the means you will have, as well as the key partners or collaborators you are going to work with.

Finally, there is the cost structure and revenue lines of your dental practice, which are located at the bottom of the model.

If you look at the image of the canvas in the Canvas model, you can see that it has some parallels with the human brain. The right side is the more emotional and creative part, from which you will create value. The left part of the model is the most logical part, where you will work on efficiency and optimization.

Following this description, it is important that you perform your own analysis. For this purpose, we provide you with a template and a description of each module. Remember:

Ideas are worthless, what counts is the ability to put them into action.

DOWNLOAD

Template 6.1: *Canvas Model*

DOWNLOAD

Template 6.2: *Canvas Model*

This graphical representation will help you reflect on all the aspects that are part of the operation of your dental practice and to make proposals for improvement.

The next step will be to analyze each block individually and see if you have a strength that you can enhance or a weakness that you should minimize.

Therefore, the canvas is not only very useful to validate your business idea or clinic, but it will also allow you to differentiate yourself from your real or potential competitors.

As you read through this book, you will understand it better, so you will probably come back to this section with clearer ideas.

Once the canvas model has been defined, you must draw conclusions to begin the innovation process, which we will discuss in the following chapters.

The business plan is drafted once the business model has been designed. This BP will give you both an external and internal analysis of your dental practice.

This document will also be your letter of introduction if you need to apply for any type of financing, either through financial institutions or investment partners.

The BP must be written and detailed. This document is neither static nor closed, as it should allow for analysis and, if necessary, reformulation or reorientation.

With this document you will have a tool to analyze your project, plan it, get to know it better by identifying its strengths and weaknesses and start it with greater coherence and rigor.

All the data obtained can be reflected in the SWOT matrix at each business moment.

At this point, you should consider the importance of having a BP for your dental practice. If you don't focus on your design, all future decisions you make will be intuitive.

The ultimate goal is for you to be able to make intelligent, data-driven decisions for better results.

Therefore, it is clear when your clinic does not have a BM and a BP, you will not have a roadmap to guide you at all times.

Scenario planning and simulations are necessary to anticipate all the possible situations you will face in the coming years.

This information will guide the strategy, which will be applied to the three dimensions that are part of this model:

People, processes and structure (PPS).

## MARKET INERTIA

In dentistry, as in other sectors, there are a number of factors that change and that you as an entrepreneur must be aware of in order to adapt your dental practice to the trends that govern the market:

- Patient profile: patients have changed, as has society and as have we ourselves. Consumer habits have evolved and their needs and demands are different from those of patients who visited a dental practice in previous years.
- Digitalization: we are in the digital era, and this entails a series of implications that will have an impact on the way you will operate and how you will communicate with the market and with your patients, both potential and current.
- Globalization: our focus can no longer be limited to our immediate environment (neighborhood), but rather we must broaden our scope of action.
- Technological progress: in our industry, technology has evolved rapidly. This provides, on the one hand, improved diagnostic and therapeutic accuracy and, on the other hand, the need for continuous updating.
- Saturation: the supply-demand balance has become unbalanced in recent years, so that competition between dental practices has increased.
- Competition: new business models, such as insurance companies or franchises, have entered our sector and coexist with traditional clinics.
- Therefore, knowing the past, present and future of dentistry —i.e., where we are headed— will allow you to stay one step ahead.

WATCH

Video Francesco Mangani:
*The door to a new dentistry*

A market analysis will allow you to understand the environment and trends, as well as the behaviors, habits and needs of the market segment you are targeting, in order to offer services that adapt and adjust to their requirements and preferences.

Although there are specialized companies that carry out exhaustive market studies, we believe the dentist, as the project leader, should be aware of these strategic aspects and reflect on them. Thus, you will be able to correctly guide and delegate the specific tasks corresponding to each business decision.

1 2 3 4 5 6 7 result

Reading time: 8 min

# The Decalogue of Success: the 10 Keys to the M_CONCEPT Model

At this point, having completed the first chapter and knowing where you are starting from (strategy), we are going to tell you where we are going through the keys that will help you achieve success with the management model.

In this book we are taking a step-by-step journey through the working philosophy, fundamentals and practical aspects of the M_CONCEPT model.

It is important to understand that for this model to be effective, it must be implemented in an orderly, comprehensive and progressive manner.

Here are the ten key aspects that make up the decalogue:

## >>>> THE 10 KEYS OF THE M_CONCEPT MODEL

1 A clear vision: your path to success

2 Differentiation: your competitive advantage

3 What is not measured is not improved

4 Achievements are made as a team

5 1st: self-management; 2nd: leadership

6 Preparation, training and continuous learning

7 Innovation, the key to progress

8 Excellence is an attitude

9 Patient-centered approach

10 ACT: no results without implementation

1. Before starting, take time to think about what professional or dental practice you want to be, project this idea, assess your resources, shape your business idea and be true to your vision.

   This vision must be challenging, creative and innovative. You should share it with your team members, as it will be the general frame of reference that will guide the operation and evolution of the clinic.

2. Differentiation means creating a value proposition and having a competitive advantage that is difficult for competitors to imitate.

   This differentiation will mark your work philosophy, your actions and your business decisions.

3. Decision-making requires information. Data is the most important strategic asset of your dental practice.

   The data will allow you to identify areas for improvement and opportunities, as well as to anticipate the demands of the market and your patients.

   Observing, recording, collecting and analyzing this information will help you make rigorous and objective decisions.

   If you don't measure what you do, you can't control it; if you can't control it, you can't manage it; and if you can't manage it, you can't improve it.

   In M_CONCEPT, we will perform a multidimensional external and internal data-driven analysis through the Golden Triangle.

4. The results of your dental practice depend on the team of people that comprise it.

   This model can only be implemented with a committed team motivated and involved with your dental practice. For this reason, we will dedicate a section to core, in order to assess key leadership issues and periodically evaluate their feedback.

5. You are the leader of this project, so management starts with you (self-management). Therefore, we focus on your personal growth and its impact on effective leadership.

To succeed in business, you need to develop specific competencies that enable you to be a better leader, with personal development as your foundation.

6. M_CONCEPT starts with the training and preparation of the leader and their team.

   Learning is an essential factor in a continuous improvement model. This methodology is oriented towards the personal and professional development of all team members.

   Lack of preparation creates risks and is proportional to the number of mistakes you make. To achieve excellence it is essential to learn, update, understand, anticipate and be prepared.

7. Innovation, both in management and technological models, will be the foundation for progress on which this model is based.

   To innovate and develop creative thinking, we propose broadening your perspective beyond the dental chair: *think outside the box*; i.e., get out of your clinic, learn from other sectors and extrapolate everything that helps you to create a different and unique service.

8. Excellence is achieved through continuous improvement in daily practice.

   This requires a commitment to your team and to your patients, as well as the use of a methodology allowing you to measure, detect areas for improvement and adapt to demand. This must be done throughout the entire care process (PDP).

9. The most successful companies are those that are customer-centric or, in your case, patient-centric.

   This approach will allow you to adapt to your patient's needs and expectations, thus achieving higher levels of satisfaction, loyalty and recommendation.

10. This whole model will be just a nice theory, with no results, if you do not implement it in your dental practice; in other words, you must take action!

    Sometimes, analysis leads to paralysis, so we give you the formula for its progressive implementation.

## RECAP

>>>> **Idea 1** Strategy is the basis or foundation of your dental practice (starting point).

>>>> **Idea 2** Through the business strategy tools, you should perform an external and internal analysis of your dental practice (vehicle).

>>>> **Idea 3** Putting this information into a BP document will guide you in your decision-making (route).

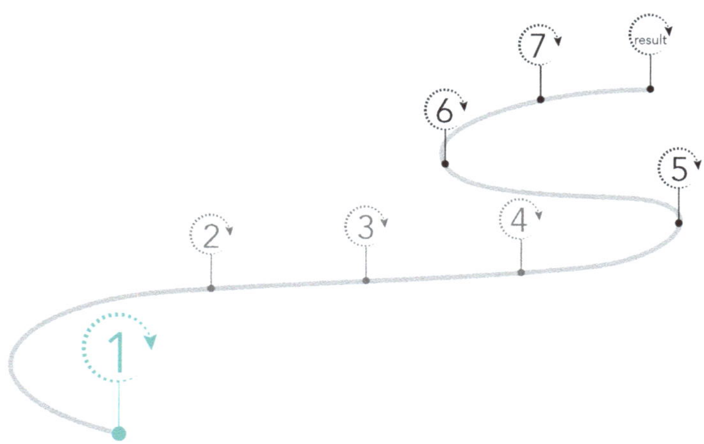

# DIFFERENTIATION

## Effective communication in dentistry

Listen to *Paspatou*,
by Parra for Cuva

Reading time:
66 minutes

Reading time: 6 min

# Everything is marketing

"Everything is marketing." The first time I heard that phrase I was sitting in a classroom at the Harvard School of Dental Medicine (HSDM) with a group of fourth-year students. My department head invited me to attend a seminar given by Fred Joyal, founder of 1-800-DENTIST and author of Everything is Marketing.

At the time, I thought: "Everything is dentistry." Why were we talking about marketing with a group of dentists and future dentists at the number 1 university in the world?

This was the moment for my first plunge into the world of marketing. I had previously read books on this matter, because it had always interested me; however, I didn't have a clear vision of its relationship to dentistry.

Weeks later I was in New York, at a fashion event organized by a magazine that a friend had invited me to and which was attended by leading international marketing professionals.

The venue was in an old restored building and all the visual elements were carefully chosen; I remember a very characteristic smell of jasmine. We were greeted by a staff person with a big smile and kindly escorted to our seats, which had signs with our names on them. Afterwards we were offered a glass of champagne and wished a happy evening.

Eight years have passed and I have not forgotten that day.

*"Products are tangible; services, intangible; and experiences, memorable."*
*Joseph Pine and James Gilmore*

In M_CONCEPT, differentiation includes the subject of communication and marketing in relation to dentistry and the strategy on which our management model is based.

The first thing you should know about marketing is its meaning. This term is often confused with advertising or sales. That is the first misconception due to which we dentists have become alienated from marketing in relation to the dental sector. Marketing is the name of a concept that analyzes the behavior of the market and its users.

The objective of marketing is to detect unsatisfied needs and design solutions to satisfy them, thereby improving people's quality of life.

There are multiple definitions for marketing. For the American Marketing Association (AMA), it "is an organizational function and a set of processes for creating, communicating and delivering value to customers and managing customer relationships in a way that benefits the entire organization."

Another relevant definition is the one described by Philip Kotler, considered the father of modern marketing, who describes it as "the social and administrative process by which groups and individuals satisfy their needs by creating and exchanging goods and services."

By the end of this book, I would like you to understand marketing as an essential element to get to know your patients and a tool for the continuous improvement of your dental practice.

Marketing allows you both to make yourself known to potential patients —i.e., those who have not yet been to the clinic (recruitment)— and to communicate with your portfolio of current patients (loyalty).

Therefore, marketing is not an advertisement or a channel or a medium, but rather a discipline that helps create value and meet the needs of patients before, during and after the care process (DCP).

In order to implement marketing in your dental practice, you must have a well-defined strategy and design a competitive value proposition. Subsequently, we will focus on coherent communication aligned with that strategy.

If you follow these steps, you will gain a competitive advantage that is impossible for your competitors to imitate.

# Communication strategies in dentistry

Reading time: 8 min

Michael Porter, a leading author on business strategy, stated that "a company can only outperform its competitors if it can establish a difference that it can maintain."

This author proposes three strategies to create competitive advantages.

The first is based on being a cost leader, i.e., offering the same service or product as the competition for a lower price, in other words, being cheaper. Regardless of whether we agree with this option, it is important to know that not all clinics can opt for this strategy. Before deciding, an economic-financial analysis should be carried out.

Some of the disadvantages of this strategy are low loyalty, since it does not build a relationship of trust with patients, and ease of imitation, i.e., it is not competitive in the face of price reductions by other clinics.

In addition, for this strategy to be viable, processes must be highly efficient and have a system in place to reduce costs, for example, in the percentages or salaries of team members or collaborators or in the purchase of materials.

The second strategy is based on being a leader in differentiation, offering something different that adds value to your product or service, for which the user will be willing to pay more. In this case, imitation by the competition will be complicated and profit margins will be higher, since the bet is aimed at doing something better and different from the competition.

The most common differentiations in the healthcare field are made through tangible and non-tangible elements: the quality of the service, the team that makes up the dental practice or the brand image, among others.

This strategy focuses on obtaining a good reputation and good positioning, which instills confidence and enables the sustainability of the dental practice in the medium and long term.

Finally, there is the focus strategy, which basically focuses on dominating a market niche, —i.e. a specific customer segment—, which can be selected according to certain variables (geographic area, sociodemographic or psychographic aspects), or focusing on a specific product/service.

This option allows for greater specialization and, therefore, a better understanding of the target at which we are aiming. Interacting with loyal patients generates higher profit margins and establishes strategies that are difficult to imitate.

The three options have advantages and disadvantages that must be evaluated, but, undoubtedly, what must be done is to define in which one to position the clinic and to have a competitive advantage, i.e., to be leaders in one of them.

Some dental practices have not defined in which of these three strategies they are positioned and, therefore, are trying to *mix* them. Thus, they abide by a management model that is not viable in the long term and convey confusing information to their patients.

When choosing a strategy in which to work, you cannot change it in the short term or mix the different options.

Imitation does not work. Competitive advantages are born precisely from asymmetries; therefore, focusing on your own strengths and not on those of the competition will be the best option.

W A T C H

Video Carlo Maria Gallucci:
*Marketing strategy*

You should avoid *me too*, i.e., positioning yourself close to the competition. This has been done in the dental sector in order to compete with large dental franchises, which is not advisable from a strategic point of view.

If you focus on your own practice, you will be faced with the so-called *blue ocean strategy*, which, unlike the traditional red ocean, is not based on competing, but rather on bringing value and innovation to the market and creating new consumption spaces positioned beyond existing demand, which ensures the viability of the strategy.

To describe the blue ocean strategy, a very representative example is often given, which innovated the seemingly exploited formula for circus shows.

Cirque du Soleil emerged at a time of crisis and changed the business model by focusing on a new type of demand (adult spectators, in addition to children), increasing the artistic value and eliminating elements considered essential until then (animals).

This business model made its competitors irrelevant and brought an innovative proposition to their field.

Therefore, remember that differences from the competition are transformed into competitive advantages (if you know how to define them).

> *"The only sustainable competitive advantage comes from out-innovating the competition."*
>
> *James Morse*

If your positioning is similar to that of your competition, you should analyze their gaps, or unmet needs, to position yourself differently than them.

You should not compete under the rules of other clinics; you should set your own rules of the game.

The competitive advantage you choose must be distinctive, profitable and communicable, among other criteria. At this point, you should reflect: Why do your patients choose you?

- Because of price? Because of the location of your clinic?
- Because of you? Because of your team?
- Because of your diagnostic and therapeutic means?
- Because of the experience they will have in your clinic?

To work on your competitive advantage you must reflect on the needs, preferences and motivations of your patients, as well as the solutions you provide, the way you do it (DCP) and the way you relate to them (communication).

The resources of a dental practice are divided into tangible (physical assets and financial resources) and intangible (reputation, etc.).

Over the years, tangible elements lose their value as a competitive advantage, as they are easily identifiable by the competition.

Technical attributes are also more easily imitable by our competitors (unless you have a patent).

However, emotionally based differentiation is complex to imitate (you, the people who are part of your team, the experience in your clinic, the corporate culture you have established, and the values that govern your day-to-day life...).

Ideally, you should combine both technical or rational and emotional aspects.

If your patients do not perceive a difference between your clinic and the competition, the decisive factor will be price. Guy Kawasaki said: "In the end, either you are different or you are cheap."

In our model we use a combination focused on differentiation through the creation and design of experiences that are perceived as unique by patients along with innovative elements that will help improve their relationship and communication with the dental practice.

It is important to know your competitive advantage. If not, you must find it and define it before starting specific communication actions. Therefore, choose your strategy and define a plan of action.

Remember: strategy is based on applying strengths over weaknesses to improve opportunities.

1 2 3 4 5 6 7 result

Reading time: 10 min

# The value proposition

*"Price is what you pay and value is what you get."*
*Warren Buffett*

Providing services without adding value is a short-term bet. The value proposition is the arguments, reasons or advantages that a dental practice has over others and that must be transmitted objectively and directly to patients.

The value proposition materializes the clinic's strategy for the customer-patient segment. This proposition must offer solutions to patients' problems and meet their needs.

Defining a good value proposition is the first step to show how your practice can efficiently satisfy a niche market.

Price is the easiest variable to modify in order to be competitive; however, few clinics analyze whether it is a cost-effective option or if it is aligned with their strategy.

In this book we want to present you with an alternative:

Bringing high added value to your service.

This is a concept that brings together the additional characteristics or values of a service and helps the patient during the process of selecting a dental practice.

Providing more value means more work, but also greater benefits. This is related to differentiation, which, in turn, is the reason why they choose you and not your competition. Differentiation will make it easier for your potential patients to choose. If you are the same as your competition, the deciding factor will be price.

A skill or knowledge that provides value to a market implies an economic value, but how much? It depends on some factors such as quality, scarcity, exclusivity, urgency, market size, competition…

A value proposition must answer three questions: *Which customer-patients are you going to target? What needs will you satisfy? What price will you set for it?*

Using the unique value proposition (UPV) we will determine three important elements: relevance, measurable value and differentiation.

This UPV is the benefit demonstrated by our clinic, which makes it stand out from the competition. The unique value proposition should be a functionality that highlights benefits that are meaningful to patients.

The value proposition is based on patient and their perceptions; therefore, in this model we will focus on them, in order to gather ongoing information that will allow us to increase the added value.

Did you know that more than 80% of customers would be willing to pay more if they were assured a better experience?

Your dental practice: *Does it have a value proposition? What distinctive activities do you perform to support your value proposition? What competitive advantage do you have over your competition?*

To determine this proposition you should not focus on yourself ("I do the best surgeries"), but on your patient ("my patient is scared of me").

*"Wonder what your customer really wants?*
*Ask. Don't tell."*
*Lisa Stone*

If you do not have this value proposition defined and tested (assessed by your target), you will be limited to a mere economic transaction and, in that case, price will again become the decisive factor.

For the value equation to be balanced, you must provide excellent service and patients must get results; this trade-off must be mutually beneficial (win to win). If the cost to the patient is higher, but they get the same results, you should focus on providing more value.

Resorting to the pricing game involves a cost that you must calculate in advance. Profit margins are only compensated if volume is high (remember that care delivery is finite, as it depends on resources such as time).

Therefore, to execute this action, analyze its profitability, assess if it is aligned with your strategy and evaluate what may affect other factors such as the quality of your service, your professional reputation...

Although this strategy is contrary to the M_CONCEPT philosophy, we do not intend to limit you or offer you an absolute truth. It will be you, with knowledge and tools at your disposal, who will evaluate, analyze and choose the value proposition you want to implement. Just remember to be consistent!

To find opportunities in the market you can reposition your service offering or your target audience, since, when the market is focused on the same customer, supply exceeds demand and differentiation efforts become more complex.

The challenge lies in understanding the unmet needs of potential patients, designing tailored services and knowing how to communicate them effectively.

*"The aim of marketing is to know and understand the customer so well that the product or service fits him and sells itself."*
*Peter Drucker*

Knowing patients better will be the best strategy for creating value. Designing an empathy map allows you to understand patients' problems, needs and desires (patient persona).

To do this, you will need to develop a semi-fictional representation of your ideal patient, whether current or potential, that incorporates all relevant information.

DOWNLOAD

Template 7: *Patient persona*

Based on this valuable information, you will design your communication, work on value creation and schedule your patients' experience in the clinic (patient experience management).

In addition to collecting information, it is very important to recognize patient profiles in order to anticipate and adapt to them to adjust the experience in the dental practice.

There are different tools to do this. The DISC method will help you assess your patients' behavior and adjust care during the DCP.

DOWNLOAD

Template 8: *DISC*

In this regard, we recommend specific training —both for you and your team—, with tests and protocols that assign the care guidelines for each patient profile.

Patient-orientation (patient centric) is the best bet a clinic can make to achieve a sustainable competitive advantage and add value.

Communication is key. Once you have defined your value proposition, you must be able to convey it correctly, through a clear and direct message. Remember: each message must be consistent with the established strategy and with what you want to communicate.

We are in the digital era and communication has changed. To contact potential and current patients we can use different channels or media; your choice will depend on your niche market and their consumption habits.

For example, on a web page they can learn many aspects about our clinic, and with the emerging social media trend we can even interact in real time.

In addition, it is possible to establish periodic communication (e.g., monthly newsletter) with topics of interest, in which to promote healthy habits, publish news about the clinic, etc.

This communication must be ongoing and bidirectional, since the value proposition will be adapted to patients' needs.

The value proposition is involved not only in acquiring new patients, but also in building a solid and lasting relationship with existing patients (engagement).

Therefore, once this proposition has been defined, you should focus on two aspects of your communication: first, that it is focused on your target audience and, second, that it is clear, attractive and direct.

Subsequently, the patient must verify that the promise is fulfilled, i.e., that they receive that differential factor that provides value.

Reading time: 18 min

# Patient Centric Model: patient focus

*"Instead of focusing on the competition, focus on the customer."*
*Scott Cook*

The patient must be at the center of your strategy and actions. Knowing your patient better will allow you to adapt and improve the DCP. To do this, let's look at it from their perspective, not yours or your clinic's perspective.

Providing services, as opposed to selling products, involves a very important characteristic, which is intangibility. Therefore, dental care can be considered an experience, in which the patient interacts with all the elements of the clinic and gains a series of perceptions, which may be below, equivalent to or exceed their previous expectations.

Therefore, in M_CONCEPT we analyze all the elements that will interact with the three dimensions we have established: people, processes and system (PPS). Based on this, perception will be shaped and satisfaction will be determined.

These elements can be as diverse as the treatment received, the smell of the clinic or the waiting time. Therefore, you must integrate them into a model that allows you to monitor and analyze them.

Your patient's perception is a critical point, as it will determine how they will feel during the care process, and this will determine their choice between your clinic or the competition.

*"People will forget what you said, what you did, but they will never forget how you made them feel."*
*Maya Angelou*

Perception is related to the degree of satisfaction and this, in turn, to the degree of recommendation and loyalty.

An analysis of the patient's path, from the moment they feel the need to the moment they search, compare, contact, visit the dental practice and repeat-recommend (loyalty process) is a key exercise.

At MBA dental® we have designed the patient journey (PJ), a tool that allows us to easily and quickly visualize the critical points and processes that take place from the moment the potential patient feels a need until they acquire our services, as well as their subsequent behavior.

To define our target audience (the one we are going to address) we carry out segmentation. To get to know and understand this segment better, we will use tools such as the empathy map and the patient persona.

The decision to go to the dentist is considered highly involved, i.e., it requires a longer process of reflection and analysis (your health is at stake, an economic investment...). Expectations in this decision are very high, as it usually involves a significant effort for the patient.

In order to provide excellent patient care, in M_CONCEPT we have adapted CRM (Customer Relationship Management) to PRM (Patient Relationship Management), which is the methodology that will help us manage the relationship with our potential and current patients.

## AIDA

To better understand the process by which the consumer makes the decision to contract a service, we will describe it through the AIDA model, which refers to the phases of attraction, interest, desire and action.

First of all, there must be a need (problem that could be solved with your services) and they must be aware of it. For example, a patient may have a dental problem, but, if it does not bother them, they may not consider making an appointment.

Pain is the term used to describe the need, concern or motivation that a patient persona has and that it can be solved with your service. If you understand the pain your ideal patient has, you will learn something very valuable: their driver or the motivation that drives them to make the decision to come to your clinic.

Subsequently, the patient must have references to your clinic; i.e., they must know you and know that you exist so that they can consider the possibility of coming to your clinic. This relates to the visibility of your clinic.

If the patient is already aware of your existence, they make a comparison and analyze alternatives, i.e., they place you in front of the competition.

Patients evaluate the best option for their needs and which dental practice will provide the solution to their problems. This has to do with the positioning of your clinic.

Finally, the patient makes a decision and takes action, i.e., goes to the dental practice. Patients choose the clinic they will visit with confidence that it will meet their expectations and solve their problems.

WATCH

Video Fred Joyal: *Two important concepts in dental marketing*

The more you are present in this process and the more you facilitate each step, the more likely you are to be chosen.

Again, the more defined your strategy and visibility, the lower the comparison will be; i.e., you will have better positioning that will make the potential patient come to you when faced with a dental problem.

Getting to know your patient and how they perceive your care process will be an area to which we will dedicate time.

DOWNLOAD

Template 9: *AIDA*

Although there are different patient profiles, in general, people who come to a clinic are increasingly more informed (or, sometimes, misinformed if they have sought or consulted information from unreliable sources), have little time, are usually more committed to their treatment and are also more demanding. The latter is something we should consider, because it will be related to their expectations.

The Patient Journey Map (PJM) is a tool that will allow you to better understand the care process. As you go through all the interactions between the patient and the clinic, you will be able to analyze areas for improvement.

Its design follows the time line from the moment the patient feels the need to the moment they come to the dental practice and leave (PDP). This involves a previous interaction (phone call, digital contact —web, social media...—) and a second phase: face to face (on-site).

*"You never get a second chance to make a good first impression."*
*Oscar Wilde*

*Moments of truth* (MOT) or *touchpoints* are interactions between the patient and the clinic that shape the patient's experience (which you will assess through the PSS items).

With the results of the satisfaction survey you can analyze whether these interactions are positive, negative or neutral. In our model, we establish positive interactions as having a Net Promoter Score (NPS): over 9.

- MOT (+): occurs when the patient is positively impressed, which has a great impact on reputation and the level of recommendation (patient promoters).
- MOT (-): occurs when patients' expectations are not met, which seriously affects the profitability and reputation of our clinic (detractor patients).
- MOT neutrals: entail stagnation, i.e., patients who come to solve a problem, but who will not recommend you and will not be loyal (passive patients).

When designing the PJM you should identify all areas for improvement. This way, you will be able to evaluate the care process step by step based on objective parameters.

The PJM will be linear at first, but then you will design it to be circular, as the loyal patient returns to the dental practice after the first visit and completes the cycle.

This map serves to diagnose the patient's experience in an orderly fashion. This information will be very useful to improve your care process and to design an innovative experience based on the data provided by your patients.

DOWNLOAD

Template 10: *Patient Journey Map (PJM)*

## PATIENT EXPERIENCE

Experts assert that most of our daily actions are guided by our subconscious. Remember the following:

Going to the dentist is also an experience.

If the patient has not felt pain or discomfort (except for aesthetic treatments that allow them to evaluate the result), they are usually left with the sum of their perceptions while at the dental practice.

Patient experience management is based on the analysis and scheduling of a unique experience at the dental practice.

To do this, you should focus on activating positive emotions during the DCP. The strategic objective allows us to consolidate a differential competitive advantage over the competition.

To emphasize the importance of emotions and experience in customer bonding, Philip Kotler used to say that brands no longer compete for market share, but for heart share.

*"Brands that succeed in generating unforgettable experiences for their customers will be stronger and more competitive."*
*Philip Kotler*

Did you know that approximately 95% of purchasing decisions are made based on emotions? Including dentist selection.

With the above statement in mind, it makes sense for dentists to have a basic understanding of how, why and what factors are involved in a patient's decision-making before they come to our practice.

Moreover, in a market as competitive as the one we are in, understanding and working on the experience is a way to differentiate you from other clinics.

Aspects such as a well-performed treatment or a price proportional to the service offered will satisfy patients' rational side, while an excellent experience will satisfy the emotional side.

If this is the case, why not start changing the messages aimed to potential patients and why not work to make their visit a more pleasant experience?

Let's take it a step further: focus on the importance of perception and stimulate your patient's senses.

**DO NOT** forget:

For the experience in your dental practice to be optimal, it must meet two requirements:

1. It must be **positive**.

2. It must be **memorable**.

Therefore, your actions from now on should be aimed at meeting these two factors.

Experiential marketing, emotional marketing or engagement marketing is increasingly used by companies to reach the emotional side of the user in a much less intrusive way.

In this sense, neuromarketing is a science that investigates three key aspects: the levels of emotion, attention, and memory evoked by stimuli in the context of marketing certain products or experiences.

Bernd Schmitt, professor at Columbia University (New York), asserts that "the client will not choose the product or the service based on the equation cost-benefit, but for the experience that will be offered before the purchase and during its consumption."

Therefore, it is no longer enough to provide a good service, you have to conquer and impact with the experience, in addition to providing a solution to a problem.

Experience based marketing in dentistry focuses on patients: on stimulating their senses and triggering positive emotions and sensations throughout the care process.

I propose an experiment: read the following words:

*perfume* *coffee*

Do you know that, at this moment, just by reading these words, activity in the primary olfactory cortex of your brain is being stimulated? Imagine everything that can be achieved during a clinical experience.

There are universal perceptions and sensations that can be implemented in a dental practice.

WATCH

Video: *Universal perceptions*

In M_CONCEPT we have experts with whom we work on sensory marketing adapted to dental practices.

Clinical digitalization opens the door to a new way of diagnosing, treating and communicating with our patients.

WATCH

Video Dr. Arturo Arciniega: *The importance of communicating effectively with your patients*

These experiences must be consistent with the clinic's communication and marketing strategy, taking into account an analysis of the patients' cultural and sociological context. This will be applied in the three dimensions of the model: people, process and system (PPS).

Once the patient has already visited the dental practice, it is important that they have excellent care (satisfied patient), that they repeat (loyal patient) and that they speak well of you (referring patient). This can only be achieved by designing an excellent and unique experience.

Communication is a key factor and, again, it must be bidirectional. You should always be open to suggestions for improvement. On this aspect, your team must be involved, know the patients and treat them with enthusiasm, taking care of every detail.

The five elements that don't fail:

- Knowledge: without a doubt, technical and care knowledge will be key to offering what is really important to patients and will allow you to differentiate yourself from the competition through an optimal care model.
- Communication: good communication is as important as the previous point. If your target audience doesn't know about your work, it will never be known. On the other hand, communication with your work team and with patients is essential for their satisfaction and for your model to last over time.
- Trust: this is an essential factor; without trust you cannot build a relationship with the patient. To build trust you must, of course, have a good practice, but you must also know how to convey it to them in all forms of communication.
- Commitment: dentists have a duty to be committed to their patients, always involving themselves in professional improvement and development.
- Perseverance: as we will discuss in the following sections, success is the sum of constant efforts and a commitment to continuous improvement.

Therefore, the better the patient's experience, the greater the likelihood of exceeding their expectations and, therefore, of building patient loyalty, i.e., that they will return to your dental practice and recommend you.

# Satisfaction and loyalty

Reading time: 8 min

Providing quality service is a fundamental aspect if the objective is to build patient loyalty. Did you know that more than 60% of people make purchasing decisions based on the recommendation of a friend or family member?

Although there are different forms of advertising, you should know that in dentistry, the best marketing strategy is word-of-mouth, i.e., your referral patients. This is related to the degree of satisfaction of your current patient base and the brand projected to your potential patients.

The patient acquisition cost (PAC) is the financial investment you must make to turn a potential user into a final conversion who will purchase your service. Typically, the investment to attract a patient varies depending on the marketing strategy.

When we focus on word of mouth, this acquisition cost decreases, since it is our own (satisfied and loyal) patients who refer new patients to us.

Before we begin, let's define two terms essential to understanding patient satisfaction: expectation and perception.

Expectation is what the patient expects from the service and is influenced by prior references to the clinic.

Perception is their assessment of the service and comes from the impressions communicated by their senses.

When the patient's perception is higher than their expectations, they achieve satisfaction; otherwise, we are dealing with a patient with some degree of dissatisfaction.

We have already mentioned that dental care is a complex process that begins before the patient arrives at the clinic and in which a series of factors and resources interact, which take place both in the office and in their environment.

Thus, it is possible to measure what happens in each of them, the people who interact and the resources available for development. This simplifies analyzing and understanding them.

The patient has a series of perceptions based on tangible factors (e.g., clinic facilities) and intangible aspects, such as the service received from the team before, during and after treatment.

This perception is related to the degree of satisfaction, which, in turn, is directly related to loyalty and, therefore, to the degree of recommendation, which is a key indicator of quality of care for a dental practice.

PERCEPTION > DEGREE OF SATISFACTION > LOYALTY

The motivations for which a patient decides to come to your office are related to their needs, but also to their lifestyle, their priorities, their values, their fears... The most common mistake is to think that this is a 100% rational process, when it is really conditioned by perceptions.

Value is perceived; it is not the real value. Value corresponds to emotional appeal and the benefits patients believe they will receive in your practice.

Another key aspect is that satisfaction is not synonymous with recommendation; therefore, you must make a qualitative leap in care.

Satisfaction is not equivalent to recommendation.

For a patient to recommend your clinic, there must be a very high degree of satisfaction. In other words, they only recommend what has exceeded their expectations.

That's why you have to work so hard on your patients' expectations. To do so, it is essential to get to know them and provide them with something different that will make their experience in your clinic positive and memorable.

To know how a service is perceived and whether the quality of the service is high or not, you must objectively know what your patients think.

Different direct or indirect methods can be used for this purpose, such as interviews, complaints and suggestions systems or questionnaires, among others.

At M_CONCEPT we have designed a survey (PSS) that allows us, in real time, to determine the satisfaction of our patients and identify areas for improvement based on the quality standards we have set.

For this purpose, we rely on the following Net Promoter Score methodology, which is an indicator to measure customer loyalty and satisfaction consisting of a numerical scale with values between 0 and 10. Only patients who rate our services between 9 and 10 will be our referrers (or promoters). Those who rate our service with scores between 7 and 8 will be passive and those who rate our service with scores between 0 and 6 will be detractors.

The NPS should be above 50. This value is obtained through a simple formula that is the result of subtracting the percentage of detractors from the percentage of promoters.

SURVEY

Satisfaction survey

NPS = % OF PROMOTORS – % OF DETRACTORS = > 50

It is important to analyze our patient portfolio and our target, since the more we know about them, the easier it will be to meet and exceed their expectations.

For this purpose, we work with a design thinking tool, which will allow us to map each of the stages, interactions, channels and elements that a patient goes through during the care process (PDP).

DOWNLOAD

Template 11: *NPS*

Using relational marketing we maintain long-term, stable and lasting relationships with our patients.

The loyalty process is the key: remember that the greatest asset of traditional dental practices is their patient base. The loyalty process will increase production and, therefore, the profitability of your dental practice.

A satisfied patient is a loyal patient, i.e., a repeat patient, which increases the dental practice's turnover. A loyal patient communicates and shares their positive experiences, i.e., they recommend our dental practice, thus acting as a referrer.

It will also have a positive impact on the positioning of your clinic in the market, since a satisfied patient leaves the competition behind and positions you as an industry leader.

Therefore, investing in patient satisfaction means, in a direct way, an improvement in profitability, in addition to all indirect benefits, which we will discuss in future chapters.

As you can see, in this model we will focus on your dental practice and your competitive advantages, establishing a competitive positioning with an internal focus.

*"The competitor to be feared is one who never bothers about you at all but goes on making his own business better all the time."*
*Henry Ford*

# Your most valuable intangible asset: your personal brand

Reading time: 6 min

## PERSONAL BRANDING AND POSITIONING

Branding is the process of building a brand, the focus of which is for patients to identify and associate it with a service.

A brand is often a company's most valuable intangible asset. In the case of dentistry, except in dental franchise or insurance models, it is usually linked to personal branding.

A personal brand is related to your daily practice and could be defined as the mark you leave on other people (colleagues, patients, work team...).

And why are we interested in dentistry?

Because personal branding is related to reliability, reputation and professional prestige.

**ME®**

Your patients want to know your story, and by that we don't just mean your CV, but also why you are in this profession, what makes you different from other professionals, what your values are, how and where you have gained experience and what you are offering to the market.

Of course, at this point you should also analyze your personal MVV, which should be aligned along with the dental practice's you lead. This will bring consistency and reliability to your patients.

Even if you are the best in an area, if you are not able to communicate it effectively and reach the people who need your services, it won't do any good. Therefore, it is important, in addition to focusing on marketing the practice itself, to engage in personal marketing.

Personal branding starts with being an expert in an area of your niche market (industry benchmark), thanks to your training and professional performance, and projecting that work to others (visibility).

The more powerful your personal brand is, the more you will differentiate yourself from your competitors and the easier it will be for patients to choose you.

Creating a personal brand or label is related to positioning, i.e., to the process of getting to know and being considered by your patients, even those who have not yet been to your dental practice.

Positioning is the place that your practice or you, as a professional, occupy in the minds of your patients in relation to your competitors.

This image depends on a complex series of impressions, perceptions and even feelings. This term is closely linked to the concept of *value proposition*.

The positioning strategy consists of defining the image to be projected. It must be directed to your target audience (target), so that they understand and comprehend the competitive difference compared to other clinics or professionals.

When this positioning is not established or is not concrete, it must either be defined or repositioned, which consists of changing the place your clinic occupies in the minds of your potential patients or current inactive patients.

Differentiation is a key factor in positioning. Positioning yourself alongside the majority of dental practices does not offer any competitive advantage. Remember that all dental practices have the option to differentiate themselves by analyzing their competitive advantages in the market.

The significance of the brand is strategically associated with a multitude of factors that can be tangible and intangible. Through this process, you must stimulate a response and create an active and intense loyalty relationship between your patients and your brand. The best positioning is that which cannot be imitated, so you must think about what cannot be imitated in each of your clinics.

Some of the frequent mistakes that occur in the positioning process include:

- Over-positioning: occurs when more is offered than can be delivered or when the price is too high, causing potential patients to refrain from purchasing those services.
- Under-positioning: occurs when we fail to differentiate ourselves from the competition or when we are simply not known.
- Doubtful positioning: this occurs when we make implausible promises. Too low a price or uncertain guarantees usually lead to rejection due to mistrust among potential patients.
- Confusing positioning: this occurs when we do not clearly define our positioning, constantly modify it or target different market segments, which creates confusion and dilutes the positioning.

The positioning map is a simple diagram that will allow you to locate your clinic and see where it is positioned with respect to the competition, based on aspects such as quality or price.

Once the positioning strategy has been defined, you should focus on making yourself known and increasing the visibility of your clinic.

DOWNLOAD

Template 12: *Positioning map*

Reading time: 10 min

# Marketing plan for your dental practice

In our model, we work with internal marketing (work team), interactive marketing (team-patients) and external marketing (clinic-potential patients).

The marketing plan (MP) is a document in which the business objectives to be achieved in a given period of time are defined in a structured manner, detailing the strategy and actions to be taken to achieve them within the foreseen timeframe.

This MP is a project created by the management and the dental practice team itself, which will help to clearly define the strategy and draft objectives to accomplish specific actions:

Object of analysis (introduction): in this case a MP for a dental practice. In this section, the geographical and temporal scope in which it will be developed must be defined.

Strategic analysis (situation analysis): for the development of the MP, an exploratory research must be carried out both internally and on environmental aspects (i.e. external analysis).

Diagnosis of the situation (SWOT): in this section a SWOT analysis will be carried out (see chapter I).

Strategic planning (specific objectives): this process involves making decisions regarding the future of the object of analysis. This section would include setting objectives for commercial profitability; visibility and reputation; and loyalty, repetition and recommendation. The commercial objectives can be defined in terms of the volume of first visits, the number of current patients who come to the practice because of the strategy, the amount of media coverage (interviews, congresses…), etc.

Marketing strategies: businesses strategies help organize the way in which the established objectives are expected to be achieved. Some of the aspects that need to be defined include segmentation (target audience or target), positioning (image you want to have compared your competitors) and communication (both with current and potential patients). The strategy (price, focus, distinction) will be selected according to the competitive advantage.

The action program is defined in response to the following questions:

- What is to be done (action)?
- When is it going to be done (schedule)?
- Who is going to do it (responsible party)?
- What investment will be allocated to do so (budget)?

Control: in addition to implementing a MP, it is important to establish review mechanisms and evaluate it on an ongoing basis to check whether it is being carried out correctly and whether the objectives set in the short, medium and long term are being met.

Drafting the plan: in the last phase, all the information gathered in the previous sections must be drafted in detail. It is important to have the support of the entire team in its design, since their involvement is essential for achieving the objectives.

The dental practice must be clear about the objectives it is pursuing and must also be aware that a marketing plan is never based on short-term profit as a fundamental goal. Rather, it is a project that contributes to the creation of value and the optimization of the brand image with the different audiences that make up the target map designed by the dental facility.

The clinic can count on the assistance of a specialized agency to help it carry out the actions formulated in the plan. However, you are responsible for making sure that the marketing strategy is consistent with your MVV and objectives. Together you will be able to establish the contents, the target, the channel, the investment, the duration...

On the other hand, the phases of the MP may vary depending on the goal to be achieved. Here is a basic model that you can start working with.

DOWNLOAD

Template 13: *Marketing plan*

Every message you send out about your practice and your staff will contribute to shaping the expectations of its recipients (potential patients).

Consumer decisions, including about dental care, are highly emotional in nature; therefore, your messages should be well targeted, emphasize the benefits of treatments (not their features) and focus on value (not price).

Both the content and the format of any type of communication from your dental practice should be carefully considered. In addition, messages should deal with health, function, and/or aesthetics (benefits), and should avoid focusing on instruments, equipment or materials (means).

If you design an advertisement, don't offer an image of an implant or an X-ray; those are the means, not the result (which is what patients are looking for and expecting).

Can you imagine a car commercial featuring a catalytic converter? You probably don't even know what it looks like, or care, if what you're looking for is a car and you're not a car enthusiast.

It is important that our patients perceive and consider their oral health with the importance it has and place it among their priorities. Dentists are responsible for the oral health messages we send to the population.

With our treatments, we improve the health, function and aesthetics of our patients, and that means being able to change people's lives through their health, with the resulting impact on their quality of life and self-esteem.

The contents covered in this chapter are very important for a dentist and their team. At MBA dental® we offer a month-long comprehensive module. During this process, we focus on the key aspects for the development of branding, image and corporate identity, which should identify our dental practice.

All of them are designed based on the concepts we have explained above. Actions, tools and design are part of the second phase.

Every element of your clinic must be perfectly aligned with the strategy: color, logo, typography, uniform, furniture, design, advertisements...; in such a way as to reinforce your position placement.

As you will see, this perspective is not limited to a marketing plan nor to the choice of a name or corporate colors, but focuses on a comprehensive and coherent strategic plan that will allow you to define effective communication, whether you want to do it yourself or you decide to hire a company.

This area is very broad: it includes different lines of action and specific knowledge in effective communication, in all its variants, related to key processes with great impact on the DCP (patient recruitment-loyalty system, social media, clinical communication protocols, budget delivery, campaigns, loyalty program, brand image...).

If you are interested in the subject and wish to expand your knowledge, we announce that we will soon publish a specific book on marketing, oriented towards dental practices under the M_CONCEPT philosophy.

## RECAP

>>>> **Idea 1** Marketing is not selling, it's communicating.

>>>> **Idea 2** Loyalty-recommendation is the key to marketing in a dental practice.

>>>> **Idea 3** The dental practice experience must exceed patient expectations and be memorable (perceptions).

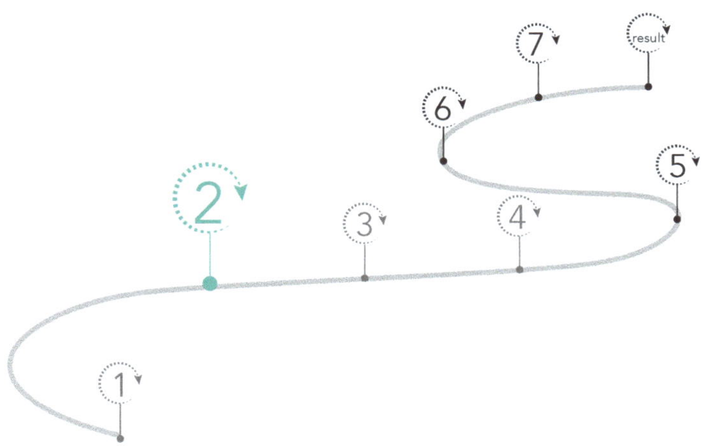

# M

the

# ANALYSIS

## The importance of measurement

Listen to *Honey*, by Moby

Reading time: 56 minutes

# M

the [illegible]

1 2 3 4 5 6 7 result

Reading time: 4 min

# What is not measured is not improved

*It was a rainy afternoon; I was on my way to the school of dentistry in Zurich. A friend had lent me an old bicycle to get around the city.*

*When I got to the traffic light, the chain came off; it started raining harder and harder. I was right in front of a coffee shop that looked very cozy, so I decided to go inside to dry off a bit and wait on the rain.*

*As I entered, a friendly waitress told me to sit at the back table, next to the heater.*

*After saying good morning, they asked me what I wanted to drink. I answered that I wanted a cafe latte. Then, the interrogation began: "Do you come here often? Are you a student? Your coffee, do you like it hot, in a large mug, powdered sugar…?"*

*Back then, it was not trendy to individualize coffee. In Cádiz they only ask you with or without milk, and they always serve it steaming hot and in a glass!*

*Seeing my puzzled look, he remarked: "Don't worry; this is just your first day! The next time you come, we'll serve your coffee to your liking, no questions asked."*

*Why did he think I would be coming back? What relevance did it have that I was a student?*

*In reality, that coffee shop wasn't the most convenient for me because of its location, but the coffee was delicious, they always had music playing in the background that brightened my mornings and the owner was charming, so I ended up going there every morning, even for Sunday brunch.*

*Years later I went back and that coffee shop still had its essence, only this time customers filled out a survey and were given a free coffee. I was very excited to recall anecdotes with the owner, to whom I told my Swiss adventures every morning. Since I left, he has opened five more coffee shops.*

*I was very pleased about this expansion. In less than two years he had structured a successful, profitable and scalable business model while maintaining the essence that characterized the original coffee shop.*

*In Zurich there were many coffee shops with delicious coffees and pleasant atmospheres. I was curious and asked: "How did you manage to multiply this business in such a short time all by yourself?"*

*The owner replied: "It's actually been years, and I did it with hundreds of people. Since I opened this small coffee shop, I have not stopped getting to know my customers in order to offer them the best service, and they are the ones who gave me this valuable information."*

Reading time: 2 min

# The importance of measurement

*"What gets measured gets improved."*
*Peter Drucker*

Measurement is improvement. To ensure the profitable growth of your dental practice, your management must be oriented towards continuous improvement; this is the basis of the M_CONCEPT model.

The use of metrics in your dental practice allows you to obtain periodic and objective information on how you are managing the resources you have; a fundamental element to evaluate, compare and improve. This translates into efficiency, as you will avoid unnecessary costs and be able to identify, correct, prevent and resolve possible errors.

Data helps us make objective decisions.

To be useful, metrics must be relevant and understandable and must be recorded periodically based on pre-standardized criteria.

Working with metrics will also be of great use in the management of the work team, as they facilitate the understanding of objectives, increase commitment-responsibility and facilitate daily decision-making.

To establish the metrics system we will differentiate four phases (MAPS): 1) Measurement, 2) analysis and interpretation of results, 3) proposals for improvement, and 4) surveillance and control.

These measurements will be based on strategic objectives and then translated into specific results (OKR system —objectives and key results—).

1 2 3 4 5 6 7 result

# The Golden Triangle: internal and external analysis of your dental practice

Reading time: 4 min

This process will be developed, both internally and externally, through the Golden Triangle.

## INTERNAL ANALYSIS

This analysis evaluates the performance and satisfaction of the work team (core); i.e. performs an internal diagnosis of the dental practice.

Performance: to implement our model you must know the key performance indicators, also called KPIs (Key Performance Indicators), and the OKR methodology (Objectives and Key Results), with which you will measure the performance of your dental practice. These KPIs will provide you with the information you need to evaluate whether you are meeting your objectives and working within the established parameters.

Work team satisfaction (core): is another aspect that you will measure. If you want to work on a total quality care model, you must take into account their satisfaction and their proposals for improvement.

This analysis makes it possible to measure the strengths and weaknesses or areas for improvement. Through this analysis you can identify your competitive advantage.

## EXTERNAL ANALYSIS

This analysis evaluates the results or final impact of your care process on your patients, translated into a high degree of satisfaction and recommendation.

Patient satisfaction: the external analysis will be based on the results obtained by your patients on the basis of the relationship between perceived quality and expected quality. With this analysis we will evaluate the *touchpoints* (moments of contact, interaction) for the three dimensions studied in M_CONCEPT: people, processes and system.

DOWNLOAD

Template 14: *Golden Triangle*

In the next phase, you will interpret the results and the surveillance-control, which we will look at in greater detail in chapter VI.

Reading time: 22 min

# Finance for non-financiers

Every business project requires an investment; therefore, you must have a financial plan. Your own-internal or outside-external sources of financing will determine the economic structure of your dental practice.

Finance is the part of economics that analyzes how funds, i.e. financial resources, are obtained and managed. Therefore, this is related to obtaining these resources (financing), as well as investing and saving them.

A dental practice is a company and therefore has economic-financial objectives:

- Generate growing and sustained revenue.
- Work with the lowest possible risk, ensuring survival and avoiding financial stress.
- Have an adequate level of liquid assets to deal with the daily activity of the dental practice.

Dentists need to have the knowledge and tools to work with a reliable financial information system.

Knowing the fundamental parameters for efficient management will allow you to make the right decisions based on objective data and gain financial control of your dental practice.

Accounting is a part of economics that allows you to get an overview of the situation of your clinic from an asset management perspective. These assets must generate sufficient cash flow to cover monthly expenses. This information is obtained through the control and registration system for expenses, revenue and other economic operations carried out in the clinic.

Accounting information must be understandable, reliable, relevant, comparable and timely. We can divide it into:

- Financial or external accounting: provides information on the clinic's equity and the results that can be obtained by using said equity.
- Management or internal accounting: costs accounting, budgets and analysis indicators.

Finance and accounting are often complex areas for a dentist, but they are absolutely necessary in this entrepreneurial process.

Our goal is not for you to be the one to carry out accounting-financial processes, but for you to understand the situation in which your dental practice finds itself (diagnosis), to be the one to make the decisions and to be able to speak the same "language" as the person or company to whom you are transferring these functions.

WATCH

Video
Dr. Ashiana Jivraj: *The importance of analysis for dentists*

Another important aspect is that business accounting is not only a tool of internal interest (for those involved in the business itself), but it is also very valuable information for external agents.

For example, financial institutions analyze, among other aspects, the financial statements of businesses to determine the viability (or lack thereof) of certain financing proposals.

To do so, we will define some basic concepts that will help you better understand the economic structure of your dental practice.

Let's start at the beginning: to record the activity of a company, accounting transactions are recorded in two documents: the journal and the general ledger.

As you know, all the daily operations that occur in your clinic are recorded in the **journal**. Each record is called a journal entry, divided into two columns: debit and credit. All entries must match in quantity (cash amount = customer amount).

Subsequently, this information is transcribed into the **general ledger**, in which each of the accounting accounts are recorded chronologically. The general ledger records the accounts throughout the fiscal year, which allows you to see trends in the accounts.

The accounts, from an accounting perspective, are expressed in the form of a T and are the basis for the accounting record of all transactions and operations that take place in the company.

The debit column includes increases in assets and decreases in liabilities, net equity and expenses, while the credit column includes decreases in assets and increases in liabilities, net equity and revenue.

Information on the clinic's equity, financial situation and income is obtained from the financial statements: the balance sheet, income statement, statement of changes in equity, annual report and cash flow statement.

## BALANCE SHEET

Is a financial document that shows the assets, liabilities and net equity of the clinic at a specific point in time.

Assets consist of goods (e.g., dental chair) and rights (e.g., patient debts). Assets must always total the same as liabilities plus net equity.

Liabilities are composed of obligations, i.e., the economic debts that the dental practice has with other companies, physical or legal persons, financial entities, suppliers, workers... Liabilities are what allow us to have asset accounts; i.e., the clinic's liabilities finance its assets.

*"An asset is something that puts money in my pocket. A liability is something that takes money out of my pocket."*

*Robert T. Kiyosaki*

Net equity is what the clinic owns (own funds) and is obtained from the difference between assets and liabilities.

Net equity = assets + rights – obligations

*Simple example of equity: we have the clinic in a premises valued at €200,000 (assets) and a bank loan (liabilities) in the amount of €40,000. The difference between assets and liabilities (200,000 - 40,000) is $160,000 (net equity).*

In the assets section, accounting accounts are arranged according to their liquidity, i.e. the possibility of converting them into cash in the short term (less than one year: current assets) and in the long term (more than one year: non-current assets).

The equity and liabilities section shows the due date of the liabilities, i.e., the maturity period of the dental practice's debts and obligations. These may be short-term (less than one year: current liabilities) or long-term (more than one year: non-current liabilities).

DOWNLOAD

Template 15: *Balance sheet*

## INCOME STATEMENT OR PROFIT AND LOSS STATEMENT

This is a financial report that shows in detail the revenue and expenses that a dental practice has had during a period of time. Therefore, unlike the balance sheet (a snapshot at a specific moment in time), the income statement shows events occurring over a given period, usually 12 months.

Revenue reflects an increase in the clinic's assets, but this does not imply that there has been an inflow of cash (collection). Revenue generates the right to receive a sum of money for providing services based on established rates.

Collection occurs when the revenue is received.

Therefore, revenue does not imply collection. Collection is the actual inflow of cash, so there will be revenue that does not materialize as collections instantly, because the patient, despite having undergone the treatment, owes that amount to the clinic.

In a dental practice, revenue comes primarily from providing services, although it may also come from interest earned on certain investments, rent, and sale of real estate owned by the company, commissions and subsidies.

Revenue is recognized in the income statement on an accrual basis (i.e. at the time the service is performed or provided, when the invoice is issued for the service provided, regardless of when the collection materializes).

Collections are recorded in the cash flow statement when the actual collection occurs.

On the other hand, for a clinic to obtain revenue, an economic effort must be made (purchase of equipment, payroll, rent, bank and insurance commissions...). All this entails a series of expenses.

An expense is not the same as a payment. An expense means a decrease in equity due to the purchase of a good or the demand for a service. It is recorded in the income statement.

On the other hand, a payment is an outflow of cash for the purchase of a good or the demand for a service. As with collections, they are recorded in the cash flow statement.

For example, we can make a purchase (expense), but not have paid the supplier (payment).

I had previously read books on this matter, because it had always interested me; however, I didn't have a clear vision of its relationship to dentistry.

We will have, therefore, transactions that refer to rights and duties: revenue-expenses (through invoices); and transactions that refer to liquid assets or cash flow: collections-payments (via transfers or cash).

The income is the figure obtained by subtracting the total expenses from the total revenue.

Revenue - expenses = income

Revenue and earnings are born from, and increased by, credit. Expenses and losses are increased by debit.

As a general rule, a company's income is calculated on an annual basis. If during this period revenue has exceeded expenses, the clinic makes a profit (positive balance). If the opposite occurs, the clinic incurs a loss (negative balance).

This analysis is fundamental, because it shows the revenue obtained by the clinic in the year in question and how this revenue has been distributed among the different expenses to arrive at a net profit, which is among the data of greatest interest.

By deferring collections over time, an additional risk is assumed that could result in definitive non-payment for the service provided. Therefore, whenever payment is deferred or installment plans are granted, it is advisable to be clear about how long and in what manner collections are deferred.

Granting installment credits can lead to the acquisition of new and more patients, which mean a higher level of revenue, which, if converted into collections, will result in higher profits for the clinic. In this case, the relationship between the risk assumed and the potential return that can be obtained must be measured.

As we can see, we are always making financial decisions that affect the future of our practice.

The financial information comprising the financial year over a period of time is reflected in the accounting cycle, which consists of three phases: opening, development and closing. It includes the financial statements, income statement, balance sheet, cash flow statement and changes in equity.

## CASH FLOW

DOWNLOAD

Template 16: *Income statement*

Cash flow is defined as all cash inflows (collections) and outflows (payments) during a given period. In other words, it is the difference between collections and payments.

*Example: if we treat a patient for €300 today, but do not get paid for 3 months, the revenue would be €300, but the cash flow would be €0.*

As you can see, right now we are not talking about revenue or an expense, now we are only including the actual inflow or outflow of cash in the clinic.

This is an indicator measuring the economic health of the dental practice and determines its capacity to generate liquidity and meet short-term obligations or debts.

Unlike net profit, this indicator takes into consideration the timing of payments and collections, thus providing a broader and more realistic view.

It is said that "cash flow is a fact, while profit is an opinion."

*Example: imagine that your clinic performs the following transactions:*

- *Treatment in the amount of €100. 20% is charged in cash (€20) and the remainder (€80) is deferred for 90 days.*
- *Purchase of material in the amount of €75. Paid in cash.*

*Income statement or profit and loss statement*

*Revenue (€100) – expenses (€75) = profit: €25*

*Cash flow*

*Collections (€20) – payments (€75) = net cash flow: –€55*

Effective liquidity management is essential to ensure the viability of your dental practice. To calculate cash flow you must take into account the profit generated, as well as provisions* and amortizations**. The formula for calculating the annual cash flow associated with the income statement would be as follows:

Cash flow = profit + depreciation + provisions

However, for a dentist, the interesting thing about cash flow (which is basically your clinic's liquid assets) is to carry out weekly/monthly control, so that you can detect a possible solvency problem in time.

Therefore, we propose the following formula:

(1) BEGINNING LIQUID ASSET BALANCE

(2) VARIATION IN OPERATING OR WORKING CASH FLOW

= + operating income – operating payments

(3) VARIATION IN INVESTMENT AND FINANCING CASH FLOW

= + other collections – other payments

ENDING LIQUID ASSET BALANCE = (1) + (2) + (3)

There are three types of cash flow: operational, investment and financing.

To ensure that you do not have solvency problems, you must have an appropriate management structure, as well as design a control mechanism and contingency plans that guarantee its existence in the event of the various situations that may arise.

Foresight is the key, because when a recovery plan is needed, it will be too late to design one.

* A provision is an accounting liability account that consists of setting aside a series of resources to meet an expected future payment obligation.

** An amortization is the decrease in value or depreciation of assets or liabilities over time.

## WORKING CAPITAL

The portion of current assets financed with permanent resources (PN + non-current liabilities) is the working capital (WC).

Working Capital indicates the clinic's ability to meet short-term payments and stay away from temporary liquidity strains.

It is a concept that you must understand, as its positive value will help ensure the continuity of your clinic and increase its profitability. Otherwise, you may encounter payment difficulties in the short term.

| |
|---|
| Working capital = current assets − current liabilities |

Positive working capital implies that current assets are greater than current liabilities; therefore, there is sufficient liquidity to assume short-term debts.

In order to balance working capital, it is important to avoid financing non-current assets with short-term debt.

Put very simply, if there are excess permanent resources to finance all non-current assets, the remaining long-term sources of financing can finance part of the current assets and avoid short-term liquidity strains.

Proper financial control, excellent expense control, the design of payment-collection terms and optimal management of the *stock*, among other measures, will help you avoid an unfavorable situation, but should you reach a negative WC, there are some options that may help you:

- Establish favorable negotiations with suppliers and banks.
- Make advance payment of collections (promissory note discounts or *factoring*): financial institutions make advance payment of patient bills.
- Offer rewards for prompt payment: this will allow you to increase sales and achieve liquidity quickly.
- Delay payments to the Government: you can request a deferral of payments to the Tax Authorities.

- Asses tax deductions (e.g., for technological innovation).

Recommendations:

- *Non-current assets should be financed with long-term debts (loans) or with capital contributed by the partners, i.e. with the permanent resources of your dental practice.*
- *Current assets can be financed with short-term debt, since this creates liquid assets, i.e., it translates into liquidity in a short period of time.*

## OPERATIONAL FINANCING NEEDS (OFN)

There are net investments necessary to cover operating expenses and perform the activity. The OFN can be calculated using the following formula:

Current assets (liquid assets + inventory + customers) - spontaneous short-term debt (suppliers)

Two metrics that give a very real view of the clinic's situation are the cash flow and the OFN.

Constant calculation and the relationship between the different metrics allow for making sound decisions based on the analysis performed.

*Do you follow me?*

WATCH

Video: *A break*

I realize that this part is complex, but remember the goal is not for you to assume sole responsibility for the finances and accounting, but to familiarize yourself with concepts to understand and interpret what the data shows about your clinic.

These parameters should not be seen as a problem, but rather as a solution that offers a wide range of possibilities you can configure.

It is useful to make complex things simple, but from a broad and comprehensive perspective of everything that happens in your clinic and that translates into numbers. Numbers don't lie!

*"We can only make good decisions if we know how to analyze and interpret the data."*

*Avinash Kaushik*

In the following section we will go into specific matters related to your dental practice.

Reading time: 8 min

# Pricing and treatment margins

The pricing strategy will depend on three fundamental factors: cost, competition and added value. In our model, competition will be less relevant.

The simplest way to set a price is to calculate it through fixed and variable costs, applying a profit margin. However, this formula does not consider the other two factors.

Before setting the price for your treatments, you must understand that this is part of your positioning, your strategy and your brand.

If you set it on a value basis, the profit margin will be higher, but you will need to have a strong competitive advantage. Remember that competitive advantage is born from internal factors. To do so, you must analyze your resources (tangible, intangible and human assets), as well as the capabilities and competencies that differentiate you.

In order to focus our strategy on generating value for the patient, it is important to know that value is what the patient receives when acquiring our service; it is what the clinic provides. The price is what the clinic receives for the sale of its services.

Before setting the price, you must differentiate the two terms described above: expense and cost, which are related to its calculation.

Expenses can be fixed or variable, operational or non-operational. The cost is the expense that the clinic incurs to provide its services.

The difference between cost and expense, in accounting terms, is that costs are considered investments that are directly identified with revenues; expenses, on the other hand, are not associated with a return on the sale of the service.

Costs and expenses are closely related, since the result of the sum of both is the production cost.

Another important aspect is to establish the profit margin, which is the difference between the price and the production cost.

The profit margin suffice not only to cover all costs, but also to help you grow. To determine this, the variable costs (VC) linked to production (electricity, water, percentage for specialists) and the fixed costs (FC) of the clinic (rent, salaries, telephone bills, internet) must be taken into account.

VCs vary in proportion to the level of activity of the clinic.

The FCs are independent of the level of activity of the clinic.

Among the VCs for our activity, there are some that are simple to obtain, for example, laboratory costs, which are clearly assigned to an activity, and others that are more complex, such as assigning to each treatment the variable cost of consumables.

They can also be classified into direct costs (DC), which are those that are clearly associated with a service, and indirect costs (IC), which cannot be clearly associated with a service, but must be distributed among different services according to some criteria. This criterioncan be units used (anesthesia), hours worked (general dentist) or any other criteria deemed appropriate.

To simplify calculations, fixed costs are considered indirect and variable costs direct, although this is not always the case. It is very important to have the exact costs of the clinic under control in order to get a real figure of the profitability of each treatment.

Understanding cost accounting will allow you to make strategic data-based decisions. This information will be useful in determining the profit margin of each treatment, eliminating or enhancing a service or setting prices, among others.

## SIMPLE METHOD FOR CALCULATING THE TREATMENT MARGIN

Direct costs (DC) are simple to identify; however, indirect costs (IC) —such as the proportionate share of electricity and rent attributed to a treatment— are more complex to calculate.

To do so, we provide you with a formula based on four steps:

1. Data collection:

   A. Number of patients seen per year

   B. Number of hours worked per year (chair hours)

   C. Total annual fixed costs

   D. Total annual consumable costs

   E. Treatment sales price

   F. Direct material cost

   G. Collaborator cost

   H. Chair hours per treatment*

   I. Number of visits per treatment

* The number of visits necessary should be taken into account. For a treatment that requires a first visit lasting thirty minutes and two subsequent visits each lasting one hour, the chair time dedicated to this treatment would be two hours and thirty minutes.

2. Calculation of cost per hour / chair (CHC)
   This figure represents the distribution of the total fixed costs among the number of hours worked per chair in the clinic.

   | CHC = C. Total fixed cost / B. Chair hours |
   |---|

3. Calculation of consumable costs / patient (CCP)

   | CCP = D. Total consumable costs / A. Number of patients served |
   |---|

**4.** Calculation of the net treatment margin*

* This is the margin the clinic has left after all costs, including indirect costs, have been deducted. To calculate the actual net margin, corporate income tax must also be subtracted.

a. With collaborator

**+ SALE PRICE**

(−) F. Direct material cost

(−) G. Collaborator cost

**= GROSS MARGIN**

(−) 2. Cost per hour/chair × No. of treatment hours

(−) 3. Consumable cost/patient × I. No. of visits

**= NET MARGIN**

b. Without collaborator

**+ SALE PRICE**

(−) F. Direct material cost

**= GROSS MARGIN**

(−) 2. Cost per hour/chair × No. of treatment hours

(−) 3. Consumable cost/patient × I. No. of visits

**= NET MARGIN**

DOWNLOAD

Template 17: *Treatment margin*

Reading time: 6 min

# Key indicators in the dental practice: Key Performance Indicators (KPIs)

KPI stands for Key Performance Indicators.

In M_CONCEPT, management by metrics forms part of the Golden Triangle analysis, which we carry out based on the objectives set according to the established strategy.

To implement a management model that ensures excellence, the performance of the dental practice must be measured on a regular basis.

These indicators will allow us to quickly identify deviations from the initial objectives and, if any, to quickly initiate a change and improvement process.

As you know, what cannot be measured cannot be controlled and, therefore, cannot be improved. Therefore, you must understand that this will be the first step to avoid "blind" or intuitive management.

KPIs are intrinsically related to the objectives, since they measure the degree to which they are being met. KPIs can be used to measure different parameters (production, quality, optimization…).

Understanding their meaning and formulation makes it possible to adapt them to the dental practice's current situation (start-up, maturity phase) and to the established objectives.

In M_CONCEPT we classify the KPIs according to the Golden Triangle and the life cycle of the dental practice.

A KPI can be a numerical figure or a percentage.

Unlike a metric, KPIs are selected because they are the key; i.e., this data helps in the making of relevant decisions for the dental practice.

These measurements must be performed continuously. In our model we establish a monthly frequency and a sustainability criterion, i.e., that stability is created on three consecutive occasions. We will also have annual metrics.

A single KPI does not provide relevant information, so in order to obtain relevant and comprehensive information about our dental practice, several KPIs must be grouped together.

The results —i.e. their calculation and graphical display— can be found in real time in the so-called *control panel.* This provides intelligent information for decision-making.

In our management model we have digitized measurements to simplify their use (one click).

In a model where we are going to continuously measure various data, it is important that it not require extra data entry work. Therefore, the data are extracted from the clinic's daily work.

With this analysis it is possible to determine the productivity of each appointment or collaborator, the average wait time, the cost per hour/chair, the percentage of loyal/non-loyal patients, the efficacy of the *recalls* system… In other words, high-value information can be gathered from each process, activity or action carried out in the dental practice.

Knowing the status of the situation allows you to take control of the clinic and act on the areas of improvement that are keeping you from your objectives. It will also allow you to detect errors and increase the performance of your daily practice.

The objectives measured by the KPIs must comply with the SMART formula:

- **S**pecific
- **M**easurable
- **A**chievable
- **R**elevant
- **T**imely, in the sense that it is possible to monitor its evolution over time

DOWNLOAD

Template 18:
KPIs

# Profitability and productivity of the dental practice

Reading time: 10 min

When we wish to analyze the economic situation of our clinic, in general, the profit is checked. This figure is not an accurate or reliable measure for calculating efficiency, since we must evaluate the amount of resources that have been necessary to obtain this profit.

Therefore, a good indicator to measure efficiency is obtained through the ratio of the profit obtained to the resources used, i.e., profitability.

To calculate it, you must analyze the income statement (profit) and the balance sheet (investment).

The economic profitability or ROA (Return on Assets) on assets measures the ratio between the profit achieved by the clinic and the value of the total assets. In other words, it measures how many euros of profitability are obtained per euro invested in assets. It is a measure of return on the quality of the investments made.

Net profit / total assets

The more the clinic's activity is optimized, the greater the economic profitability. To do so, it is necessary to:

1. Increase the number of sales (volume of treatments).

2. Increase the profit margin.

ROA is the basic indicator for evaluating efficiency in business management and is expressed as a percentage.

Financial profitability or ROE (Return on Equity) is not tied to total operations, but to those derived from the own funds. Refers to the return obtained per euro of net equity.

Net profit / own funds

ROE is therefore the ratio between the net profit obtained by the clinic and the capital invested by the partners. In other words, it is the partners' profit related to the money they have invested in the company.

To improve financial profits, the dental practice can opt for debt, provided the economic profits are higher than the cost of external financing. This is called financial leverage.

ROE does not include the debt ratio and ROA does not take into account sources of financing, which is why they are usually compared in order to establish the company's real profitability situation.

Yields occur when the clinic's total revenue exceed total expenses.

The break-even point is the one where the clinic begins to generate a profit.

The higher the revenue and lower the expenses, the faster the profit threshold will be reached.

Which treatments bring the greatest profit to your dental practice?

This is of utmost importance that you perform this analysis. To do so, you must determine which treatments are the most profitable.

In some clinics, the Pareto rule is followed, which indicates that 20% of the treatments bring 80% of the profit.

To do this, you should always work with tools that allow you to determine the profitsof each treatment and apply the RICE matrix (Chapter V).

## PRODUCTIVITY

Productivity is the measure of the value you produce (output) with the resources you use (input).

Productivity = output/input

To increase productivity you can focus on the following strategies:

- Increase value (output) with existing resources: this translates into differences in the value proposition.
- Decrease resources (input) to generate the same: this refers to process efficiency.
- Work on both strategies.

In M_CONCEPT both strategies are addressed.

A ratio that will help you understand your dental practice is:

Productivity = production/work time

Productive work time regarding to clinic presence time is the effective presence.

Effective presence = mouth work/presence in clinic

Productivity refers to measuring the efficiency of the production process in your dental practice. Some related factors are organizational, technical, personal and related to production, among others.

Simplification and standardization of the care process are directly related to the productivity of the dental practice.

In this sense, management is the key. Having an efficient method that allows you to coordinate your work team and optimize resources will increase your clinic's productivity.

Therefore, the goal is to produce more with less. In the following chapters you will see how excellence and innovation will provide you with the necessary mechanisms to increase productivity through value proposition and process optimization.

When your dental practice begins to generate a profit, one aspect you must consider for steady and sustainable growth to occur is reinvestment.

In our M_CONCEPT model, reinvestment is a very important factor that is analyzed in relation to the strategy.

Your dental practice is a motor that requires continuous investment. The best time to reinvest is when the accounts figures are positive.

Therefore, you raise the pay out when you obtain a net profit, i.e., distribute it among the partners or reinvest in order to grow the dental practice. Reinvestment would be included in the company's net equity as reserves.

## RECAP

>>>> **Idea 1** Measurement is the only way to improve.

>>>> **Idea 2** The balance sheet, income statement and cash flow statement are the accounting documents that help you make better decisions.

>>>> **Idea 3** The performance of your dental practice is based on objectives that are measured with key performance indicators (KPIs).

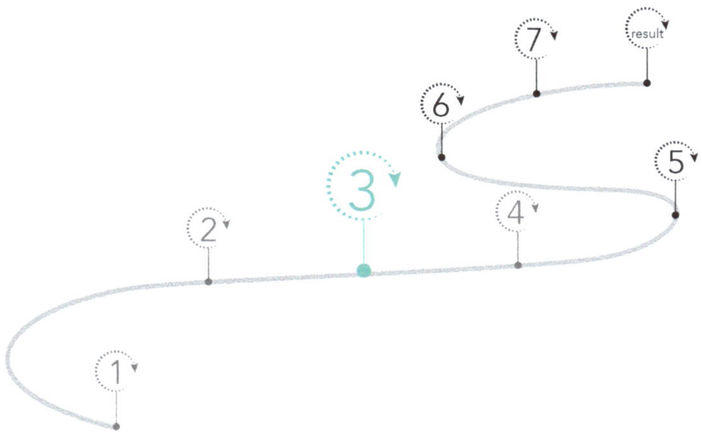

# CORE

## Your dental practice's greatest asset

Listen to *Man o to,*
de Nu

76 min

Reading time:
76 minutes

# M

the book

1 2 3 4 5 6 7 result

Reading time: 2 min

# It's all about teamwork

*One of my first international flights was to England. I still remember feeling uncertain and excited at the same time.*

*That summer I decided to immerse myself in an experience to improve my English along with two Spanish friends. During those months, we worked in a hotel serving breakfast.*

*It was a small hotel, with that characteristic British charm, where the same guests came every summer for long stays during their vacations.*

*Most of the customers were retired and they were really nice to us, especially when we didn't understand a word of what they were asking!*

*One day, a guest asked us: "What's wrong with you guys?" to which, dumbfounded, I replied: "Excuse me, I didn't quite understand you." "Yes, normally you are always smiling and clearing the tables together, today was not like that."*

*Indeed, the day before, we had a discussion to agree on whom should clear the tables and, therefore, finish later, in addition to doing the chores that nobody wanted to do: picking up trash, cleaning the kitchen…*

*This gentleman was a retired businessman with whom I had daily conversations. Since our manager was not there that day, I shared my dissatisfaction with him.*

*When I explained the situation to him, after a smile, he remarked: "Why don't you work in a rotation and change positions every day? That way, you will all finish sooner and share the work that no one wants to do."*

*It's all about organization, it's all about teamwork!*

# Corporate culture

Reading time: 20 min

*"Management is the development of people and not the direction of things."*

*Lawrence A. Appley*

Your work team, your greatest asset. The people who are part of your team are the heart and engine that drive your dental practice.

Some authors call them internal customers. The same is true for providers and all those who make the daily clinical work possible. They are a fundamental element in our management model: core = nucleus.

In M_CONCEPT we focus on developing high performance teams.

Proper team management and the creation of a good work environment are the necessary framework for improving satisfaction, productivity and performance.

If you don't take care of your team, you will lose their motivation, commitment and involvement.

Designing a satisfying and productive work environment is a major challenge facing most dentists.

Excellent service is the result of coordinated and interdependent work by the team of people who are part of a dental practice.

Investment in personnel, including salaries and benefits, translates into high operational costs. This means that any factor influencing their ability to work should be considered a priority issue.

When our students start at MBA dental®, their initial concern is focused on the area of finance or quality of care. As they go through the program, they tell us that team management is the most complex part of the program for them.

Unlike certain indicators, which can be calculated with predictable formulas, people are different, so there is no single equation that allows for the effective management of all team members.

However, you can (and, from our perspective, should) train yourself to be a better leader, achieve an optimal work environment and obtain well-being, satisfaction and, therefore, higher performance from your work team.

Your commitment as a leader is to establish a management model that is sensitive to the needs of your employees and to achieve alignment between your team and the vision of the dental practice.

In M_CONCEPT this is a key pillar, evaluated periodically through the Golden Triangle.

Your team's degree of satisfaction and all suggestions, observations and proposals for improvement must be continuously compiled and analyzed.

Today, compensation is an important factor, but not the only element valued by employees. Other considerations such as work climate, flexibility, and means of conciliation or personal-professional development are criteria that determine the choice and satisfaction of the people who form part of a team.

The core, in most dental practices, is usually small. Even so, it is necessary to acquire skills that enable the leader to manage it correctly and make each person feel motivated and committed to their functions.

The work environment has a direct influence on the degree of satisfaction and motivation of the team and, therefore, on the performance of the clinic.

In order to design a suitable environment, it is essential for you to understand the meaning of corporate culture. Before implementing it, let's define it: "Corporate culture is your team's overall way of thinking, feeling and acting that identifies the clinic to patients, collaborators and providers." It could be described as the "personality" of a company.

Every dental practice must have an identity, standards and principles of action.

Some authors indicate that there are three levels to this concept (De Long and Fahey; Edgar Schein):

- First level: values, which are the essence of culture, the basic beliefs that determine the behavior of each individual. These are the most difficult aspects to learn and modify.
- Second level: norms, based on values and easier to perceive. They determine the correct behavior of the organization.
- Third level: practices, which translate into the most visible and easiest aspects to identify and modify.

In function of focus, there are three different classifications for corporate culture. One of the classics is by Cameron and Quinn (based on the *Competing Values Framework*), in which they differentiate between four types:

- Clan culture: its focus is internal; teamwork, commitment and involvement are encouraged.
- Hierarchical culture: its focus is internal; control, standardization, process standardization and efficiency are encouraged.
- Adhocratic culture: its focus is external; creativity, risk-taking and initiative are encouraged.
- Market culture: its focus is external; it promotes the achievement of objectives, internal-external competitiveness and productivity.

Other authors, such as Roger Harrison (*Harvard Business Review*), define them according to business objectives and the values associated with them and classify them into four orientations:

- Power-oriented organizations.

DOWNLOAD

Template 19: *Types of corporate culture*

- Standard-oriented organizations.
- People-oriented organizations.
- Results-oriented organizations.

According to organizational culture expert Carolyn Taylor, there are five cultural archetypes in companies: innovative culture, achievement culture, unique team culture, customer-centric culture and people-centric culture.

The current trend is to focus on results and people, with a flexible approach.

Corporate culture translates into everything you do on a day-to-day basis: the way decisions are made, communication, how resources are organized...

This, together with knowledge, is part of the intangible resources of your clinic and is what differentiates you from others; in other words, the culture of an organization is consolidated as a competitive advantage.

Therefore, it is something you must define to reinforce your strategy.

## THE CULTURE OF YOUR DENTAL PRACTICE IN 5 STEPS

To define the culture of your dental practice, we suggest you establish the following phases:

1. Define in writing the corporate culture you want in your dental practice based on your MVV.
2. Diagnose the current situation.
3. Describe and share with your team the values, behaviors and norms, in function of the culture, that you want to implement.
4. Establish consistency between what you think, what you communicate and what you do and evaluate your consistency in your daily operations.
5. Involve the team in the corporate culture (appropriate selection of profiles and integration of the corporate culture).

Successful organizations are characterized by strong cultures that attract, retain and build team loyalty.

To design a high-performance team, the first step is to define, identify and manage human talent. To this end, we will establish four phases: selection, training, compensation and evaluation.

## SELECTION OF THE WORK TEAM: COMPETENCIES AND CULTURAL FIT

Selecting the right team is the starting point. Therefore, your ability to choose the right people will be the first step in forming the core of your dental practice.

*"An intelligent person hires people who are more intelligent than he is."*

*Robert T. Kiyosaki*

In this selection, it is important to evaluate two aspects of their background:

- Functional adjustment: analyze the technical skills (hard skills) of the candidate to ensure that they are in line with what the clinic needs (training, competencies, experience, etc.). This information is usually obtained through their CV. It is easy to evaluate.
- Cultural fit: evaluate other transversal skills (soft skills) and the candidate's alignment with the clinic's culture. Communication skills, teamwork are evaluated... This aspect can be examined during the interview phase.

The hard skills open a door for the interview and the soft skills determine job position.

To have the right team, i.e., one providingthe right mix of aptitudes and attitudes, you should draft the profile characteristics before the selection process.

*Recommendations: hire slowly, select the best profile.*
*This will prevent staff turnover and increase performance from the start.*
*Surround yourself with talented people.*

## TRAINING

Invest resources in training your team. A good leader is capable of recognizing the abilities of each team member and enhancing them, i.e., obtaining maximum performance.

Talent is the most important variable in any organization, which is why we must focus on the ongoing education and training of each team member.

Personal development is a very important motivating factor. The team must grow at the same pace as the clinic.

## TRAINING, DEVELOPMENT AND OBJECTIVES (TDO) PLAN

Training is related to the clinic's strategic plan and objectives. To do so, we will define the objectives for each position or profile. These individual objectives should be aligned with those of the clinic and should be measured through the corresponding KPIs.

To meet these objectives, you must design a development plan, i.e., train and empower your team to facilitate their achievement. This will be established through an initial meeting and, subsequently, feedback will be obtained through follow-up meetings (every three months) and a final evaluation meeting.

In our model, the TDO plan will be reviewed annually to adapt it to the established needs-objectives and to consider the results obtained in the surveys (ESC).

The training program will not just focus on technical knowledge; to this end, training must be expanded and oriented towards improving the areas in which deficiencies are identified (e.g., communication skills).

The SWOT analysis of the Golden Triangle will guide you on the areas for improvement towards which you should direct your investment in training your team.

## COMPENSATION

The company's compensation policy is one of the factors that influence the level of team satisfaction. The compensation plan is a fundamental aspect that must be defined for each profile or role.

There are different types of compensation:

- Fixed compensation: is established based on the functions or position, with a minimum fixed by law, and adapted according to the market reference. When it is established on the basis of the professional competencies and characteristics of the person occupying the job, it is called individualized.
- Variable compensation: is established based on results or achievements. These are set through objectives (strategic and operational) and measured through KPIs.
- Flexible compensation or compensation in kind: this type of compensation supplements the base salary or variable compensation with non-monetary benefits (e.g., vacation days, flexible hours, training…). Compensation in kind is not allowed as the sole salary compensation, so it is usually combined with the other two types of compensation: fixed or variable.

This system favors work-life balance, improves the company's image, offers tax advantages and adapts to the needs of each individual.

The compensation system you design must be in line with your strategy and must be simple, fair and transparent.

In the case of freelancers, you must establish an office rental contract or a service lease contract. Billing would be done directly by the worker to their patients.

In addition to individual competition and incentives, you can establish bonuses, which are extraordinary payments that depend on the overall income, i.e. that achieved by the work team as a whole.

It is important that your team's perspective reach beyond the next payroll.

Salary = financial compensation + emotional salary

> *Important note: the emotional salary (work climate, personal development, shared MVV, conciliation…) is what motivates your employees or collaborators; the economic remuneration is the compensation for the work done (what they take for granted).*

In addition to the employment contract, we are going to introduce the term emotional contract. According to Juan José Goñi Zabala, there are elements related to the capabilities of organizations that depend on intangible factors such as the motivation, participation and commitment of people to business projects. In this sense, he proposes five levels of emotional contract.

## EVALUATION: PERFORMANCE AND SATISFACTION OF THE WORK TEAM

Analyzing the performance and assessing the evolution of your team are necessary functions for the continuous improvement of your dental practice. Defining criteria for measuring performance and stimulating its constant improvement is an effective system for achieving objectives.

In our model, we will do this through KPIs and OKRs (Objectives and Key Results), that will be assigned for each profile or *role*, enabling it to be results oriented rather than task oriented.

The main function of OKRs is to connect the individual objectives of each employee to the clinic's mission and to achieve measurable results. This will help keep each team member motivated and involved.

In management by objectives, we focus on achieving, not on doing. Each task must be oriented to the achievement of previously established objectives.

We will also evaluate the team's own satisfaction, through the ESC (Golden Triangle), consisting of four dimensions (motivation and recognition, organization, area and work environment and finally training/professional development + open questions and proposals for improvement).

In this way, we will obtain the feedback necessary to understand the current situation, make adjustments, proposals for improvement and face new challenges.

1 2 3 4 5 6 7 result

Reading time: 6 min

# Leadership in dentistry

*"There are leaders and there are those who lead. Leaders hold a position of power or influence. Those who lead inspire us."*
*Simon Sinek*

Most dentists are required to form a work team, so they serve as leaders in administrative and managerial functions.

In this chapter we will address personal leadership through self-awareness and leadership applied to your team and your dental practice.

Is a leader born or made? I'm sure you have heard this question on several occasions and have asked yourself.

The reality is that some people have an innate ability to assume the role of leader, something inherent to their personality. However, most people need to learn, train and experiment to become good leaders.

Some studies have shown that around 24% of leadership skills have a genetic component, so the remaining 76% can be learned and developed (*Initiative One Leadership*).

Everyone who leads work teams takes on a great challenge. Therefore, if we want to have a high-performance team, we must be trained in this subject.

Motivation, communication and decision-making will be tailored to the specific situation we will be leading.

There are three variables related to leadership type: the characteristics of the leader, the characteristics of the work team and situational characteristics.

*"If your actions inspire others to dream, learn more, do more and achieve more, then you are a leader."*
*John Adams*

Leadership style influences the team, since the leader's behavior generates motivational mechanisms that have a great impact on the behavior of each member.

There are multiple classifications of leadership styles. Those classically described revolve around three dimensions: participative, collaborative and instrumental leadership styles.

The participative leadership style is characterized by a leader who considers the opinion of the team and involves it. In the collaborative style, the leader tends to be helpful and focuses on the well-being of the group. Finally, instrumental leadership is characterized by a leader who proposes and decides how to carry out the team's functions, defining standards and work methodologies without consulting the team members.

The managerial grid of Blake and Mouton is a leadership model that identifies the degree to which a leader focuses on people or task-results.

DOWNLOAD

Template 20:
*Types of leadership*

Another broader classification describes the following styles: *laissez-faire*, democratic, autocratic, transactional and transformational.

One style is likely to predominate in a leader, although this does not mean that, in a given context, there cannot be combinations.

DOWNLOAD

Template 21:
*Management Grid*

In this regard, Paul Hersey and Ken Blanchard designed the situational leadership model and a tool (LEAD) that allows leadership to be tailored according to the maturity level of the team members and the situation.

It is important that you know each style, firstly, because you will feel more identified with one of them and, secondly, because you will have to analyze the type of leadership that best fits your strategy and the current needs of the dental practice.

DOWNLOAD

Template 22: *Types of leadership 2*

From M_CONCEPT we have selected those characteristics that we consider essential to achieve a quality care and team satisfaction model (variables that we are going to measure).

1. Team involvement (MVV defined).
2. Importance of two-way communication.
3. Promoting professional development and talent retention.
4. Focusing on results (through structured processes).
5. Commitment and motivation (team satisfaction).

DOWNLOAD

Template 23: *Situational leadership*

The leadership style must encompass both rational and emotional factors. Remember that the right hemisphere (emotional and creative) and the left hemisphere (rational and deductive) are involved in this relationship.

Reading time: 12 min

# Team satisfaction: motivation and engagement

*"Coming together is a beginning. Staying together is progress. Working together is success."*

*Henry Ford*

The satisfaction of your team is one of the key parameters for the success of your dental practice. For this reason, in our model, it is one of the pillars of the Golden Triangle.

Motivation is defined as the drive and effort to satisfy a desire or fulfill a goal. Satisfaction is experienced when the result has been obtained. People's behavior is oriented towards the satisfaction of needs and the achievement of their objectives or aspirations. Motivation consists of those factors capable of provoking, maintaining and directing behavior towards these objectives. Motivation is the factor that determines the productivity and performance of the work team, so we will analyze its meaning and impact.

First of all, let's explain a related term: *self-concept*. Self-concept is the opinion a person has about themselves; i.e., the way they feel, think and see themselves in relation to their environment. This drives behavior, performance and results.

Self-concept consists of three components:

- **Ideal:** is what we aspire to be (dreams, goals).
- **Self-image:** is the mental image or representation we have of ourselves, influenced by the treatment we receive from our environment.
- **Self-esteem:** is the core of the self-concept, the opinion one has of oneself. It determines energy, enthusiasm, vitality and confidence.

When these three aspects are taken care of, motivation increases and team members feel respected, valued and important. As a result, performance increases exponentially.

For your dental practice to be a high-performance organization, you must create a high self-esteem environment for each person on your team.

Motivation can be intrinsic or extrinsic. Extrinsic motivation is due to external factors and the motivated behavior is carried out in order to achieve something (rewards). Intrinsic motivation is based on internal factors (needs, interests, curiosity, and satisfaction) which drive long-term sustainable productivity.

Initiatives to increase team commitment and productivity are usually based on external rewards (salary increase, flexible working hours…), which have a short-term effect and are limited, i.e., they end when the reward is removed. Internal motivators (feeling valued, self-fulfillment, finding purpose and meaning in their work) achieve deeper engagement and are sustainable over time.

Based on these premises and understanding the concept of *motivation*, you will be able to establish effective strategies for each member of your team.

*"Outstanding leaders go out of their way to boost the self-esteem of their personnel. If people believe in themselves, it's amazing what they can accomplish."*

*Sam Walton*

There is no exact formula for motivating a work team. Motivation is related to priorities, life stages, interests and hobbies, as well as the personality type of each member.

The key is to understand the people who are part of the team and to understand the link between the effort-performance, performance-results and results-satisfaction of individual objectives.

Getting the team to contribute their best guarantees success in the process of continuous improvement at the clinic. To do so, three requirements must be met:

- To want: to have determined intention to participate in continuous improvement.
- To know: to adequately channel the team's knowledge towards continuous improvement. To do so, they must be committed to patient satisfaction (know what to improve) and have the necessary training to be able to improve processes (know how to improve).
- To be able: implementing continuous improvement requires an investment in resources, so it is necessary to provide our team with everything necessary for its implementation.

In a company or organization, it is important to know how management influences success-failure. According to the attribution theory of Lee Ross of Stanford University, when an individual achieves success, they attribute it to their own merit; however, when they fail, they attribute it to the system. People, when they feel they are failing, disconnect from the organization (in this case, from their responsibilities to the clinic), while when they succeed they connect, become motivated and involved.

Engagement is a term used in the field of organizational culture that is identified with voluntary effort on the part of workers. An *engaged* person is involved and enthusiastic about their work, and a high degree of motivation is essential for this.

If our team feels committed to the clinic, they will be willing to make additional efforts and thus produce good performance, such as performing above and beyond what is required of them, taking on new responsibilities and providing great value.

This philosophy can be incorporated from the outset, i.e. during the selection process through job crafting, which consists of adapting the job position according to the candidate's skills and objectives.

There is a positive correlation between engagement and performance improvement beyond the conventional performance-based approach. Today's professional profiles no longer focus on work as a means to cover their basic economic needs, but rather aim to find personal fulfillment in the performance of their professional activity. Therefore, they seek to develop their professional interests and the motivation that will allow them to exploit their talents.

Having common goals and a roadmap for where you are headed will create a climate of confidence that will ultimately translate to your patients.

Another important aspect is recognition, which means communicating and letting the team know that the clinic appreciates and values their work and effort. Recognition is an aspect that generates feelings of belonging to the organization, group feeling, motivation so as to work and make an effort. This also enhances individual and group self-esteem.

## >>>> THE 5 GOLDEN RULES FOR BUILDING A HIGH-PERFORMANCE TEAM

### 1 Spend time with the people who are part of your team

For your team to function in a coordinated manner, you must know each profile perfectly. Treat your team as what they are: your "corporate family;" that way, they will feel safe, comfortable and motivated.

Promote team relationships by organizing meetings and periodic afterwork sessions.

### 2 Involve your team in the why, in addition to explaining the what and the how

Understanding the why, makes them participants in the project and aligns them with the strategy, increasing their degree of involvement. The likelihood that objectives will be achieved will be greater if each member is convinced of the value of their performance and if they perceive that their actions will effectively contribute to achieving them. In addition, the why, the reason your clinic works every day, will be a determining competitive factor that will generate great value and will be almost impossible to imitate.

### 3 Create an environment based on respect and communication

It is essential to establish relationships based on respect in a work team, and this starts with your approach to leadership. Knowing the opinion and understanding the experience of your team increases the value they perceive, allows you to improve processes and, in addition, helps your dental practice to be more competitive. Communication is the difference between management and leadership.

### 4 Value the qualities of each member of your team and support their growth and development

Encouraging the personal-professional development of your team, valuing those challenges that make them feel recognized, will create a more competitive environment in which performance and productivity will be higher. To give our team autonomy in performing their functions, to delegate and to trust them, they must be empowered. To do so, establish an annual training program according to the needs of your clinic and team. With innovative and visionary leadership you will identify opportunities for improvement and design an environment that stimulates creativity.

Training in M_CONCEPT is an indispensable requirement, as it will allow us to work in a continuous improvement model and adapt to new changes and challenges.

### 5 Create successful experiences through attainable objectives

Setting achievable goals (OKR system), sharing the clinic's vision, providing clear guidelines and recognizing achievements form the basis of a successful environment.

Setting goals according to each person's level of experience and ability encourages a winning attitude. When objectives are achieved, you should acknowledge them both privately and publicly and provide a reward tailored to the needs and expectations of each team member. Subsequently, you should set new objectives that represent new challenges to achieve, for which the team will commit to continue advancing in the established strategy. This will give them the opportunity to feel a sense of accomplishment in their daily work. If these goals are not achieved, try to break them down into smaller, more attainable goals. Remember that our model involves progressive implementation.

*"Happiness is the secret ingredient for successful businesses. If you have a happy company it will be invincible."*
*Richard Branson*

Working with a satisfied team will increase your clinic's performance and decrease staff turnover, creating a synergistic environment for the clinic and your patients.

The basic purpose will be to create a good working environment that will have a positive impact on the operation of the clinic and result in excellent patient care.

Remember the following phrase:

*"Happiness is productivity."*
*José L. Fuentes*

Reading time: 6 min

# Communication

*"The art of effective listening is essential to clear communication, and clear communication is necessary to management success."*
*James Cash Penney*

Knowing how to communicate is an essential skill in business. Establishing a transparent, clear and concise communication system will improve the organization and have a great impact on work environment.

Your communication is related to the way you think and act. As Luis M. Díaz-Meco says: "Be, do and —only then— communicate."

To maintain consistency, before establishing a communication system, you must go back to the first chapter, i.e., develop a defined strategy, since it will determine the way you will communicate (with the team, with current and potential patients, with suppliers…).

## INTERNAL COMMUNICATION

Internal communication is that established within the dental practice. It can be carried out in either a formal or informal context. The latter tends to focus primarily on interpersonal relationships and is often the one that has the greatest impact on well-being at work.

It can also be defined as vertical communication (ascending or descending), between leader and employee, or horizontal, which occurs between individuals who have the same position or job.

These aspects will determine the how, i.e., they will determine how communication is adapted to each context.

Establishing a two-way internal communication system (leader-team) facilitates coordination and the exchange of opinions, increases the degree of motivation, reduces the number of errors and allows you to measure the "pulse of your practice" through the perceptions of your team.

*"The art of communication is the language of leadership."*
*James Humes*

When we talk about communication, we also refer to practicing active listening, receiving feedback from the team and writing down all their suggestions, ideas and contributions.

In our model we work on the rules that regulate communication in the dental practice, i.e., the communication protocol.

In this protocol, the messages, the channel (medium through which they are transmitted) and the receivers must be specified.

Some essential ingredients for establishing effective communication are empathy, i.e., the ability to put yourself in the other person's shoes, and assertiveness, which is the ability to express your point of view while respecting that of others.

*"The verbal component of a face-to-face conversation is less than 35% and over 65% of communication is done non-verbally."*
*Mehrabian*

You have probably heard about Albert Mehrabian's 55-38-7 rule, which states that 7% of communication potential is based on verbal language (words); 55% on body language; and 38% on paraverbal language or use of the voice. Therefore, non-verbal communication accounts for 93% of communication.

With these data, you can assess the relevance of both verbal and non-verbal language and the need for dentists to be trained in this subject. Through an effective communication system, you will increase the productivity and efficiency of your clinic.

Persuasion is a term that, *a priori*, has been associated with a certain negative connotation as it is associated with the manipulation of opinions, ideas and people. I hope that, after this introduction, you will be able to "unlearn" its meaning in order to integrate it correctly. In our model this becomes important because, through persuasive communication, we are going to improve the attitudes of our team and our patients. This is an acquired skill.

Paul Watzlawick said that it is impossible not to communicate. Every act of voluntary communication involves persuasion, even in everyday activities.

Persuasion is the use of communication to change, shape or reinforce people's attitudes. This is essential in organizations.

*"If you can't communicate and talk to other people and get across your ideas, you're giving up your potential."*

*Warren Buffett*

In this sense, your approach should always be focused on benefiting your team and patients.

Persuasion is also based on two fundamental pillars that you must work on every day: credibility and trust.

In addition, you must show consistency between what you think, what you do and what you say.

*"Example is not the main thing in influencing others. It is the only thing."*

*Albert Schweitzer*

## EXTERNAL COMMUNICATION

External communication is directed at potential and current patients, as described in Chapter II (in M_CONCEPT: differentiation).

# Organization chart

Reading time: 6 min

The clinic's management must extract the activities from the strategic plan and define responsibilities, delegate tasks and provide the necessary means for their execution.

The organization chart is a visual representation of the relationships and functions that are established in the dental practice. It is a system that identifies the workflow and how team members are grouped around it.

Organizational structure is a key aspect of our management model, as it is related to process optimization. Delineating this organizational structure is essential so that each team member knows the tasks to be performed and also to avoid confusion, friction and reduced productivity. This will allow for efficient coordination between the people-process dimensions and ensure optimization of the care process.

Each person needs to know exactly what is expected of them and how their contribution will be evaluated against the clinic's objectives. The team must be involved in the detection of errors and in the development of proposals for improvement.

Organizational structures can be classified as functional, divisional, matrix and project-oriented. A dental practice is usually structured by function. Setting up the internal organization of the clinic is part of the strategic process.

In M_CONCEPT we propose a process management approach (PMA), so the graphical representation of a process will transversely cross the clinic's organization chart and will be result-oriented. Thus, the objectives will be aligned with the needs and expectations of the patients, without strictly adhering to the classic functional relationships. Processes must be well defined and documented, with the responsibilities of each member clearly identified and a responsible person assigned.

Therefore, we will adopt a horizontal organizational chart concept (activities or processes), different from the traditional "vertical" organization (departments or functions). We propose that you design a complex (strategic) chart and another simple (operational) organizational chart.

To design the strategic organizational chart, the first step is to define each role, which will be assigned a code. The information you should complete for each role includes:

- Mission: role and objectives in the dental practice.
- Description of specific tasks-functions-responsibilities.
- Requirements for the position: education, specific knowledge, skills, work experience-type profile.
- Training to be provided to new team members.
- Availability: workdays and schedules.
- Documentation: information handled and generated.
- Remuneration: salary.
- Skills: professional or personal attitudes required (hard & soft skills).

This template can be modified and adapted to the needs of your dental practice and its use is limited to people who manage strategic processes.

The operational organizational chart, however, contains less information, but it should be available and placed in a visible place so that anyone on the team can refer to it. This template includes tasks-functions and workdays-schedules.

The roles and responsibilities of each profile must be accepted by the responsible member. To do this, we recommend that you draw up a document with all the information they need to know according to their *role*.

> *Recommendation: take time to get to know each role: its functions, its environment, the resources available to it (materials, time…), etc. "Rotate" through each job, this will help you understand it better and integrate it into the care process.*

Albert Einstein said: "Example isn't another way to teach, it is the only way to teach." This phrase takes on special meaning when talking about the relationship between a leader and their team.

Design a welcome plan to facilitate the integration and adjustment of each new team member. Organization is a fundamental aspect that will mark the efficiency of your dental practice.

When you implement M_CONCEPT in your dental practice, you will see how the structured workflow makes for accurate timing, adherence to schedules and minimized errors. This will create productive workdays, which should be combined with moments of relaxation and disconnection.

Reading time: 24 min

# Self-management: area for personal growth

*"You cannot manage other people unless you manage yourself first."*

*Peter Drucker*

Talking about entrepreneurship without addressing the personal side is practically impossible. Personal growth is the basis for entrepreneurship.

You are going to be the person who inspires a team. Train yourself, prepare yourself and work on the competencies that will allow you to be a good leader.

*"Before you are a leader, success is all about growing yourself. When you become a leader, success is all about growing others."*

*Jack Welch*

I am sure that, simply by taking the time to read this book, you are already a professional with an interest in learning and improving and, therefore, a restless person, with high expectations for self-improvement.

Personal and professional goals are often closely linked. That is why we will dedicate this section to reflecting on some aspects related to the personal side.

The balance between emotions, mind and health will influence your entrepreneurial attitude.

*"Self-assessment is the first action required of leadership."*

*Peter Drucker*

Self-awareness is the result of a reflective process through which we acquire a notion of our personality, capabilities, competencies, skills, abilities, interests and possibilities. It is an exercise that brings us closer to knowing our potential and positions us in relation to our strengths and weaknesses.

A good leader detects their weaknesses, surrounds themselves with people to help them overcome them and empowers their team.

According to Daniel Goleman, self-awareness means having a deep understanding of our emotions, strengths, weaknesses, needs and motivations.

It is important for you to stop at this point and define your personality, as it will be the basis for marking your weaknesses and strengths, which will be related to leadership.

To help you get to know your personality better, we suggest you perform the following exercise:

TEST

Discover your personality type

## GET OUT OF YOUR COMFORT ZONE AND TAKE ACTION

All entrepreneurship involves stepping out of our comfort zone, taking risks and exploring new horizons. The challenges in the initial phase are accompanied by insecurities and fear of failure (you've probably had that feeling).

However, to achieve goals, overcome challenges and fulfill dreams you must take action. Once you have overcome that barrier, you will find the learning zone, the growth zone and, finally, the realization zone (cross & grow).

As you already know this path, now you just need to take the step; the first one is the most complicated, but you have to take it, even if you are afraid.

Get ready, surround yourself with the right people and jump in.

Transform your projects into actions.

*"Someone's intelligence can be measured by the quantity of uncertainties that he can bear."*

*Immanuel Kant*

## LET'S TALK ABOUT FAILURE

In the business world, people talk about success formulas, but it is very important that you know the other side of the coin: failure. Failure is not achieving the intended result. Fear of failure is often the main obstacle on the road to a goal.

*"The greatest mistake you can make in life is to be continually fearing you will make one."*

*Elbert Hubbard*

From our perspective, failure is an essential element of success. It is an ingredient for any major achievement. Fear of failure is conditioned by three factors: the interpretation of a situation, the anticipation of possible consequences and the evaluation of the result obtained.

Why is failure important? One of the main reasons is that during this process, if you know how to deal with it correctly, there will be a learning process that you will extract to use on future occasions.

It is very likely that, on your entrepreneurial journey, you will encounter obstacles and make mistakes; it is part of the equation for change, progress and business sustainability. Therefore, knowing how to integrate them and being prepared will help you develop skills such as: developing responses to problems, adapting to adverse situations or reacting quickly.

Believe it or not, these situations often bring out our greatest potential. Failure is an excellent opportunity to move forward. It strengthens our resilience and stimulates creativity to design alternatives and solutions.

Our personality and behavior influence the way we manage failure. True failure is persisting in the same mistake or giving up in the face of an unforeseen obstacle. Failure is combated with learning, analysis and perseverance.

Preventing or minimizing failures and identifying the most frequent causes of a clinic's failure to succeed are somethings we will focus on. Therefore, we need to understand our mistakes, analyze them and draw up an improvement plan. As David Kelley said: "Fail faster, succeed sooner."

One important aspect is that, if you work in an analysis and continuous improvement model, you will make "micro-errors," which are easy to detect and fix. It is essential to have a defined SWOT analysis and an action plan, which will help you face new challenges.

*"Great leaders are not defined by the absence of weakness, but rather by the presence of clear strengths."*
*John Zenger*

## EFFICIENT PEOPLE

Return on time invested is a way of analyzing the benefits of your efforts. Income can be earned in three main ways: time-based income, performance-based income and passive income.

A dentist, with their clinical activity, mainly produces benefits from an effort made over a period of time. For that reason, you must measure your efficiency and organize your schedule, as time is finite. In addition, the more efficient you are, the more time you can get out of your schedule to achieve a work-life balance.

A simple tool that will allow you to organize and prioritize tasks is the Eisenhower matrix.

DOWNLOAD

Template 24: *Eisenhower Matrix*

## ENTREPRENEURIAL ATTITUDE: ARE YOU A REACTIVE OR A PROACTIVE PERSON?

As mentioned earlier, attitude is extremely important in the entrepreneurial process. Your response to events or circumstances will mark your path towards your objectives.

A reactive person waits for events to happen before reacting. This is the person who is overwhelmed by adverse situations, perceives change as a threat, has little initiative and tends to blame others for their mistakes.

A proactive person is willing to take control of the situation, proposes solutions, takes responsibility for complex situations and does not wait for opportunities, but creates the circumstances for them to occur.

Which one do you feel you identify with the most?

You should work on being a proactive person, as this will help you to maintain anticipatory, change-oriented behavior and take control of the situation.

## THE POWER OF HABITS: SELF-DISCIPLINE AND COMMITMENT

Habits are the intersection between knowledge (what, why), abilities (how) and motivation (desire). These habits determine important changes in our lives.

*"I am a great believer in luck. And I find the harder I work, the more I have of it."*

*Thomas Jefferson*

Habits mark daily behavior. Napoleon Hill, in his book *Success Masters*, indicates that effectiveness is built on discipline and routine.

Most exceptional people, i.e., those who are excellent in their personal and professional performance, are so because they implement certain intellectual, emotional and operational micro-skills.

If you are interested in expanding on this topic, one author we recommend is Stephen R. Covey, who in his work *The 7 Habits of Highly Effective People* discusses the importance of habits to implement on a daily basis, which will help you achieve professional and personal accomplishments.

*"Life is but a tissue of habits."*
*Henry F. Amiel*

## CONTINUOUS LEARNING

The current context demands continuous learning. It is a fundamental value because it allows us to be in continuous renewal and growth. Incorporating new knowledge moves you away from stagnation and allows you to maximize opportunities.

Stephen R. Covey said that the most powerful investment we can make in life is to invest in ourselves.

Self-investment in training is one of the best decisions you can make. To be an excellent practitioner, your training should not focus exclusively on technical or dental-specific training. Focusing on acquiring new skills will enrich your personal and professional development.

## THE IMPORTANCE OF NETWORKING

A proper connection to your environment can accelerate and boost your career path. Connecting with people is a way to create alliances and build projects to achieve common goals.

Sometimes, networking is related to large companies or other areas outside of dentistry. Dentists and dental practices must foster our network of contacts with providers, colleagues, patients, partners… Having a good network of contacts will enhance our professional career and the positioning of our dental practice.

Did you know there is a theory that states, using a mathematical formula, we are connected to anyone in the world by no more than five intermediary contacts? This is the theory of the six degrees, which was developed by Frigyes Karinthy.

Develop and take care of your networking, and not just in the dental field!

## WORK-LIFE BALANCE

To be productive you must maintain healthy habits. Your mental, emotional and physical health is directly related to your potential.

High-performing individuals need to work on their work-life balance, i.e., the balance between professional and personal life.

You must establish this balance in your personal life and in that of your work team. This contributes to quality of life and makes it possible to harmonize professional development with personal objectives. To this end, it establishes a conciliation strategy, with specific actions. An emotional salary brings satisfaction, productivity and stability to the workforce.

## THE FORMULA FOR SUCCESS

The factors that determine success have been researched for years. The RAE (Real Academia Española [Royal Spanish Academy]) defines *success* as the "happy result of a business, performance, etc."

Although we will start from this statement, the definition of success has a personal and subjective component and will depend on the perspective from which we approach it. Establishing an effective algorithm for success in a constantly changing environment is difficult. Even so, here are some of the formulas that have been defined regarding business success.

According to the University of Illinois, the formula for success depends on three variables:

$$S = 3D$$

*S = success; D1 = desire; D2 = determination; D3 = discipline.*

Ricardo Ros, in his book *La fórmula matemática del éxito* [The mathematical formula for success], highlights above all the attitude with which we face situations.

$$S = [(I + A2)(P \times F)]_D$$

*S = success; I = idea; A2 = action now; P = persistence; F = flexibility; D = diversion.*

Victor Küppers also highlights the importance of attitude in what he defines as the "attitude effect," meaning the sum of knowledge and skills multiplied by attitude.

$$V = (K + S) \times A$$

*V = value as a person; K = knowledge; S = skills; A = attitude.*

According to Eric Hoffer, the formula is based on the following variables:

$$S = (ID + DP) \times EA + P$$

*S = success; ID = inner desires; DP = direction or purpose; EA = effective action; P = persistence.*

Albert László-Barabási adds that success is not individual, but communal, so it is not focused exclusively on you and your performance, but on how others perceive your performance. The collective definition of success requires thinking about how your work impacts other people. We suggest you read about this author, his formula for success and its relationship to networking.

$$S = Qr$$

*S = success; Q = a person's ability to execute an idea or combination of talent and innate ability; r= value of the idea.*

The road to success is based on small daily improvements that bring you closer to your goals. There is a formula that states that small daily progress (+1%), accumulated day after day, and translates into exponential growth.

$$1.01^{365} = 37.8$$

In M_CONCEPT we are going to propose an open definition, in which you are going to choose its meaning, extending its implication beyond making the right decisions in a business environment.

In all formulas there are always three elements for the chain reaction to success: a substrate (skill, talent...), a spark that triggers the start (desire, idea...) and an essential component, oxygen (perseverance, discipline...). In the recipe for success, you are the one who adds the ingredients, and the proportion will depend on the value each of them has for you.

W A T C H

Video Fernando Botella:
*Ingredients of success*

## >>>> THE 10 ASPECTS THAT DEFINE AN ENTREPRENEUR

Entrepreneurship is comprised of a series of abilities, attitudes, values and ways of acting. We have selected those personal factors and motivations that we consider necessary in an entrepreneurial profile:

What makes the difference:

1 PASSION: is the engine that drives the action and gives meaning to the undertaking.

2 VISION: is to project into the future, identifying a strategy for success that others do not see, and charting the path to achieve it.

3 CREATIVITY: is the talent to generate new ideas, concepts or associations that produce innovative solutions.

4 AUTHENTICITY: is a value that makes a person inimitable. To act with authenticity requires self-awareness and self-management.

A must-have:

5 PERSEVERANCE: is the virtue of remaining consistent, even when circumstances are adverse and in spite of failures.

6 DETERMINATION: is the ability to make decisions and solve problems, meeting objectives effectively; always through prior analysis.

7 TRAINING AND PREPARATION: entrepreneurs face great challenges that require multidisciplinary training, so training will be the basis on which the entrepreneurial process will be developed.

What helps you progress:

8 FLEXIBILITY: is the ability to adapt to circumstances and react to changes; in environments such as the current one (VUCA) it is an essential factor.

9 TEAMWORK AND EMPATHY: the ability to relate appropriately with the people in the environment is a key factor; the team multiplies the results.

10 COMMUNICATION: being able to convey opinions, ideas, feelings or information effectively is a must for an entrepreneur.

This combination is composed of innate factors and factors that can be acquired. The entrepreneurial process involves continuous learning, which comes from preparation or training and associated experiences. The pace and manner of learning is up to you.

## RECAP

>>>> **Idea 1** The core is the engine and the heart of your dental practice.

>>>> **Idea 2** To have a high-performance team, you need their motivation, involvement and commitment.

>>>> **Idea 3** Before success comes attitude.

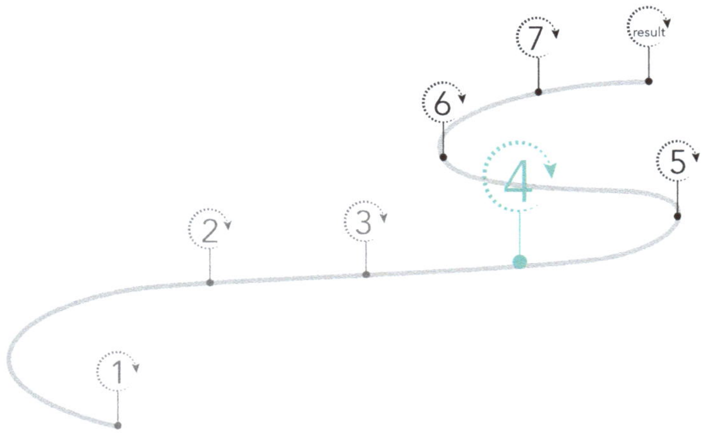

# INNOVATION

## The key to progress

Listen to *Versailles (hold)*, by Christian Löffler

36 min

Reading time: 36 minutes

# M

the [illegible]

1 2 3 4 5 6 7 result

Reading time: 2 min

# Innovating is thinking differently

*Four years ago, I was the director of the Dental Research Group (Grupo de Investigación en Odontología, GIO) and a member of the Miguel de Cervantes European University's ethics committee. My duties included reviewing research projects submitted to the Health Sciences Department.*

*An expert in genetics presented us with a study focused on nutrition and sports performance. Meanwhile, a team of engineers was developing software capable of detecting and simulating the movements per millisecond of facial mimicry, for the design of animations.*

*In the cafeteria where we used to meet once a week, two mathematics professors showed me a prototype that made it easier for people with mobility restrictions to use instruments.*

*Eleven months later we founded Dental Genetics®, a company that uses the analysis of DNA from the cells of the mucous membrane of the mouth and saliva to diagnose systemic and oral pathologies. Fourteen months later, we developed facial analysis software that allowed us to obtain real-time information on the patient's hard and soft tissues.*

*Fifteen months later, after developing a brush prototype (*HTB brush*) with a pneumatic system, we received the University-Business Award for enabling people with restricted mobility to use instruments that allow them to autonomously perform everyday actions, such as eating or brushing their teeth.*

*Innovating is bringing value to people in a different way than before.*

# Innovation process in the dental practice

Reading time: 6 min

*"Every person, institution, company or society to survive needs to learn, at least, at the speed at which the environment changes."*
*José Antonio Marina*

Innovation and excellence are the basis for our management model, M_CONCEPT. Through innovation, your dental practice can grow and position itself as a market leader.

One of the definitions of the term *innovation* pertains to Professor Michael Schrage of the Massachusetts Institute of Technology (MIT), who defines it as "the conversion of novelty into value."

In a VUCA environment, adaptation is the key factor. Flexibility and quick learning, coupled with the ability to take action, will be the best tools for the advancement of your dental practice. Adapting to changes in the environment means evolving.

Innovation is synonymous with producing, assimilating and successfully exploiting a novelty, in such a way that it provides new solutions to problems and makes it possible to respond to people's needs.

Innovation is a process that can modify what already exists or create something new that has a favorable impact on the market. Therefore, it can be achieved through improvements, and not just the creation of something completely new.

It can be implemented progressively or rapidly. We can therefore speak of disruptive innovation or incremental or adaptive innovation, when it is carried out gradually.

*"To innovate is to use knowledge, and generate it if necessary, to create products, services or processes, which are new for the company, or to improve existing ones, thus achieving success in the market."*
*Oslo Manual (1997)*

From the M_CONCEPT perspective, innovating is providing answers to problems or needs (present or latent) by developing new value propositions (*market-pull*) adapted to the needs of the market.

In other words, solving problems (pains) and seizing opportunities (gains).

When we talk about innovation, we not only focus on technology; we can also innovate in the management model. A different approach will allow us to distance ourselves from our competitors and adapt to an increasingly changing and competitive market.

Innovation is change, improvement and progress.

The innovation process must be cost-effective and sustainable and always be patient-oriented.

Innovation brings competitive advantages. The survival and success of dental practices will depend on their competitiveness, which in turn will depend on their ability to innovate and adapt their services.

Innovate or disappear

The market is demand-driven, so finding differentiating factors that increase demand will determine the growth of your practice.

The degree of innovation in our processes and services has a positive influence on their return on investment. This culture of innovation must be integrated into the strategic objectives of our dental practice.

According to Alfons Cornella, innovation consists of generating ideas that are perceived as valuable, so as to produce sustainable results. The equation is:

$$\text{ideas} \times \text{value} = \text{results}$$

In M_CONCEPT, innovation means generating new ideas, implementing them in our service, improving processes, providing value to our patients and increasing profitability.

Therefore, innovation is about growth, profitability and differentiation of the dental practice.

To innovate in your clinic, you must align your strategy and your team to this process. To do this, it must be systematized and oriented to specific results. Some clinics focus on a particular type, but the opportunities for improvement multiply when multiple innovation processes are explored.

Therefore, innovation is a key pillar of any clinic that plans to grow in the short and long term.

## TYPES OF INNOVATION

As we have mentioned, innovation is not just about incorporating new technologies. To this end, we are going to describe other types of innovation that must be combined for the innovative process to be effective in our dental practice:

- Innovation in the structure: brings together innovations related to the organizational structure, the management process or the business model, among others.
- Innovation in the offer: focused on the services offered and on the actions related to the functionality of these services.
- Innovation in the experience: related to the interaction systems between patients and the work team.

1 2 3 4 5 6 7 result

Reading time: 14 min

# Innovation in the management model

When we talk about innovation in dentistry, the incorporation of new technologies probably comes to mind. In our model, we extend this concept of innovation to the management model.

To this end, we would like to introduce you to the blue ocean philosophy (*Blue Ocean Strategy*), developed by W. Chan Kim and Renée Mauborgne, professors at INSEAD (Institut Européen d'Administration des Affaires [European Institute of Business Administration]) business school and authors of the book of the same name published in 2005. This theory is based on market expansion through innovation, making competition irrelevant.

In the traditional red ocean, companies are constantly focused on their competition and exposed to the emergence of new competitors, which diminish their growth possibilities. The challenge is to outperform the competition…, sound familiar?

In contrast, in the blue ocean, companies focus on generating new demand, creating value and differentiating themselves from the competition.

In the blue ocean there is an untapped market space that will create an opportunity for profitable growth.

This represents a paradigm shift in the business focus.

Probably, if you have not heard of this theory before, you will think it sounds utopian or you will not find it applicable to your dental practice.

You should know that this is not merely a "nice theory," but is part of market-tested strategies that have been used by companies such as BMV, Ralph Lauren, Electrolux, Nintendo…

Before going into its usefulness in dentistry, let us explain the example of Cirque du Soleil, which is very simple and illustrative to describe the blue ocean strategy.

At a time when circus shows were in decline, two brothers —Gilles Ste-Croix and Guy Laliberté —managed to reinvent themselves through a new business model, with which they achieved differentiation and a reduction in costs.

This was achieved by focusing on a new type of demand and changing the classic competitive factors of the sector: adult viewers (as well as children), increased artistic value, elimination of animals from the show… With all this, they managed to offer a model that positioned their competitors on an irrelevant plane.

This was something that had not been considered, following the traditional competitive scheme, in the apparently exploited formula for circus shows.

If you focus on and extrapolate this example to your own practice, you will be presented with the so-called blue ocean strategy, which, unlike the traditional red ocean, is based not on competing, but on bringing value and innovation to the market: creating new consumption spaces, looking beyond existing demand and ensuring the viability of the strategy.

> *"If you don't have a competitive advantage, don't compete."*
> *Jack Welch*

And how are you going to do it? From a customer-patient perspective, you must analyze your positioning in the market with respect to your competitors, in order to innovate in your service. You should also consider your target audience, because you may be able to focus on "non-customers," i.e. forgotten or unserved market segments.

Your objective will be to gain a better understanding of the customer-patient segment and be able to adjust your value proposition to their expectations, aspirations, frustrations and actual needs.

## THE COMPETITION (OR NOT)

*"Make the competition irrelevant."*
*W. Chan Kim*

With our approach, you will notice that competition is analyzed as an improvement factor, a change factor and even an irrelevant factor when you succeed in working on a unique value proposition.

At M_CONCEPT we focus on innovation and process improvement as the main factors for competitiveness, to offer an experience that exceeds our patients' expectations. In other words, our efforts and attention are focused internally.

One analysis that will help us is the so-called *value curve*, which is a tool that graphically represents key values and is differentiated between: the variables most valued by patients, the scope of competitors and the position our clinic holds within the competitive framework.

## INNOVATING IS EVOLVING THE VALUE PROPOSITION

When you analyze the competitive factors of dental practices through the value curve, you will be able to see how you can distance yourself from the competition.

DOWNLOAD

Template 25: *Value curve*

If the lines trace the same position, you will be offering the same thing as the competition; therefore, you will not hold any significant competitive advantage.

Let's look at an example. W. Chan Kim, an author of reference in our program, proposes working in a space that is not exploited by the competition. The key lies in ensuring that the strategy is conceived from the patients' perception of value.

To design a value curve, you must follow these steps:

1. Define the competitive factors of the sector: the elements that your patients value most (price, quality, professionalism, accessibility, facilities, personalized attention...).
2. Identify your competitors and their value propositions.
3. Include your clinic in that chart based on competitive factors.
4. Compare with your competitors.

With the value curve you will understand how the patient perceives the market and, in addition, you can use it to understand the unserved variables that are important to users and disregard those that are not.

Point 1 can be adapted to your environment, i.e., you can ask your patients what factors they value most in a dental practice (PSS). This way, you will be able to analyze whether you fulfill them and determine your position with respect to the competition.

## THINK DIFFERENTLY

One of the objectives we have proposed with this book, as we indicated at the beginning, is to give you a different perspective so you can begin to reflect on aspects that you may not have considered before.

To innovate, it is important not to focus solely on the needs of current customer-patients, but to explore new market needs.

> *"If I had asked my customers what they wanted they would have said a faster horse."*
>
> *Henry Ford*

While it is important to improve what is already working, we invite you to think outside the box. We assure you that, comparing the dental sector with others, there is still a long way to go! Sometimes it is not necessary to invent, just extrapolate what is already being done in other companies or sectors and implement it in your dental practice.

I can tell you that innovation is the basis of all my lines of work (clinical, teaching and research) and the growth engine for every project in which I am involved.

Observe and learn from other companies, from other sectors. You can do this while traveling and getting to know a new hotel, while waiting at the dealership for your car to be delivered, at the bakery near your home... You just have to open your mind and get out of the walls of your dental practice!

In summary:

"Think outside the box."

Or our version: "Think outside the dental chair."

## THINKING ABOUT NON CUSTOMER-PATIENTS

One focus that can help you differentiate yourself is to modify your target audience, i.e. the people you are going to appeal to. Clinics usually target the same or all patient profiles, i.e. they do not segment (they do not focus their strategy).

It is also important that you analyze needs from the perspective of non-patients: What makes them "non-consumers" or what limits them from coming to the clinic? Dental fear or phobia, ignorance (they do not know the importance of correct oral health or the maintenance guidelines), lack of courage (it is not among their priorities), lack of budget...

At this point, you should turn your attention to understanding and exploring unmet needs and addressing those limitations. If you succeed, you will be entering a thriving segment in which you will be the industry benchmark.

One example is Curves gym. This gym was based on a target audience that at the time was a non-customer profile in gyms (adult women). This business model specializes in a specific segment and designs training sessions tailored to its customers, i.e., adapted to their needs.

You can also maintain your target audience and innovate in the treatments or services you offer to your patients.

Therefore, remember that identifying needs and understanding your patients sets you apart from your competition, which can be transformed into competitive advantages if you are able to think differently and broaden your perspective.

If your positioning is similar to that of your competitors, analyze the gaps or unmet needs to place yourself in a position different from that of said competition. Don't compete under others' rules; set your own rules of the game.

At this point, you should reflect:

1. Do you offer something different than your competitors?
2. What is your competitive advantage, and what is your value proposition?
3. How can you add value to your DCP?
4. Do you know your target audience?
5. How do you meet their needs?

If you go back to Chapter II, which strategy do you most identify with? Do you want to change the strategy or reinforce the current one?

*Recommendation: it is important that you answer these questions before starting specific actions. If you are not clear about them, pause, reflect and define them.*

Therefore, set your strategy and define an action plan.

## CREA MATRIX (CREATE-REDUCE-ELIMINATE-AUGMENT)

This tool allows the value proposition and the value curve or competition curve to be redesigned.

The above variables can be included in a RICE grid, in which you should consider, for your strategy, the elements you should create (C), reduce (R), eliminate (E) and augment (A).

DOWNLOAD

Template 26: *RICE grid*

This analysis will allow for value innovation.

For example, if you have a clinic that specializes in a specific area, it may be worthwhile to expand treatments or services and eliminate others that require investment and are far from your focus.

Imagine you are a pediatric dentist: maybe incorporating conscious sedation is more advantageous than keeping a prosthodontist. Or, if you are an endodontist, invest in a microscope instead of adding new offerings.

This would be an example of factors that could be increased and others that could be reduced or eliminated, reducing expenses and investing in the same line of work. This improves positioning, reputation and quality of service (super-specialization) while optimizing resources (same professionals, no need to hire new dentists).

Of course, before making this type of decision, you must analyze your strategy (MVV) and do a performance calculation (profitability of each treatment, number of treatments in each area…).

1 2 3 4 5 6 7 result

# Innovation in the patient experience

Reading time: 4 min

One of the most important ingredients in designing the patient experience in a clinic is innovation. The surprise or differential factor is only obtained if you do something new and different from the competition.

This entails a broad and creative approach. To innovate, it is necessary to know and understand patients and, of course, to be trained in this field in order to make the right decisions. Patients help design a service tailored to their needs, modeling what needs to be improved, incorporated or eliminated.

Thanks to innovation, you will be able to offer a service with elements that will allow you to impact and create memorable experiences for your patients.

In M_CONCEPT we rely on the design of a unique sensory experience that makes patients perceive a positive value in the dental practice. You already know the importance of perceptions and their impact on satisfaction.

Companies such as Apple, Ikea or Starbucks, among others, have worked along these lines, increasing the engagement of its customers beyond the product.

Sensations perceived through the senses activate our neural system and generate emotions. Remember that the dental practice experience should be positive and memorable. This design is related to attraction, differentiation, satisfaction and brand loyalty.

This experience is implemented through sensory marketing. This is not based on a creative process guided by intuition, but requires a specific methodology.

Through the PSS and CSS, you must analyze the information that is important to your patients-team and set priorities, which will guide you on the investment you will make to shape the experience. The dimensions on which you should work are formed by people-processes-structure (PPS), described by M_CONCEPT.

The temperature of your dental practice, the smell, the sound, the light, the treatment received, the design…; all these factors must be taken care of and must maintain coherence with your strategy (MVV). Each factor provides information. However, for it to be an optimal process, it must be properly planned and receive the right advice.

At MBA dental® we have experts in sensory marketing that study each case in order to create a unique DCP.

1 2 3 4 5 6 7 result

# Technological innovation

Reading time: 6 min

Technological innovation allows professionals to work with greater precision, in both diagnosis and treatment. In addition, it optimizes processes and allows for the efficient use of resources (human, material and time).

Digitization is a milestone that has changed the way patients are diagnosed and treated and has become an essential element in today's dental practices.

Therefore, we join the process known as physical-to-digital-to-physical:

- Physical to digital: information is collected from the physical environment and a digital record is created.
- Digital to digital: information is shared and interpreted using advanced analytics, analysis and artificial intelligence (AI) to interpret relevant information.
- Digital to physical: algorithms are applied to translate digital information into actions and changes in the physical environment.

We can also talk about new technologies that will be implemented in the coming years. We are facing the Fourth Industrial Revolution, also known as Industry 4.0. This revolution is changing the way companies operate and the competitive environment.

Industry 4.0 is based on the use of smart technologies that will be integrated into organizations, people and assets. As in other sectors, dentistry is making advances in robotics, analytics and big data, artificial intelligence (IA), genetics, digital dentistry, nanotechnology and the Internet of Things (IoT), among others.

WATCH

Video Ignacio Pedrinaci: *Digital dentistry*

At MBA dental® we count on the latest technologies applied to the dental practice, through the collaboration of partners and with the development of tools that make management easy.

WATCH

Video Dr. Kyle Stanley: *Artificial Intelligence applied to dentistry*

The trend is towards the ability to adjust and learn from data obtained in real time, making clinics more responsive, proactive and predictive. This will have a final impact on our patients, as it will increase the individualization of the services offered in dental practices.

## HOW DOES TECHNOLOGICAL INNOVATION BENEFIT YOUR DENTAL PRACTICE?

The implementation of new technologies in your dental practice brings direct and indirect benefits in the short, medium and long term.

If you want to take full advantage of all the benefits of the various advances, you must ensure that you have clear and measurable objectives and, above all, that you obtain useful information to be able to make decisions.

DOWNLOAD

Template 27: *Example of a decision tree*

1. Indirect/medium to long-term benefits: innovation improves the performance of the dental practice, since its incorporation has a great impact on competitiveness and adaptation to change. An innovative attitude within the clinic will make the organization more resilient and able to respond with agility to different scenarios.

2. Direct/short-term benefits:

   a. Differentiation from the competition: implementing innovative elements will positively differentiate you from the competition.

   b. Patient care: innovative solutions are focused on improving communication, experience and process automation, minimizing errors and work times. The impact on the patient's final satisfaction is one of the factors that stand out in this innovative process.

   c. Clinical quality: new techniques and technologies make it possible to obtain greater diagnostic and therapeutic precision in a faster, simpler and more predictable manner. This is the basis for minimally invasive dentistry (MID) and individualized dentistry (holistic approach).

   d. Efficiency: one of the objectives of innovation is to simplify the DCP and improve work efficiency, a factor that will have a positive impact on the clinic's profitability.

## HOW DO YOU START THE INNOVATION PROCESS IN YOUR DENTAL PRACTICE?

- Strategy: every innovation process begins with good planning, aligned with the objectives.
- Assessment: before implementing innovation, a predictive study should be carried out, including the initial investment, its ROI (return on investment) and the expected final impact.
- Integration: implementation involves a learning phase, adaptation of work protocols and the design of new processes.
- Analysis: this will be carried out by measuring the results obtained, including possible proposals for improvement.

At this point, we will work with an algorithm that allows us to design a flow for decision-making prior to investment.

Reading time: 4 min

# Investment and ROI for innovation

Investment in innovation creates efficiency, productivity, competitiveness and value. To analyze the effort made, we work with input metrics and output metrics.

The amortization of the technologies you incorporate in your dental practice must be analyzed beforehand, stipulating the impact and return on investment (ROI).

It is important to analyze different aspects during the implementation of innovation and new technology: financial, logistical and performance aspects.

Input metrics are used to measure the economic, time or talent investment dedicated to the specific activity related to innovation management. Output metrics are used to refer to the return on that investment.

## QUANTITATIVE ANALYSIS: ECONOMIC-FINANCIAL

In M_CONCEPT we divide the investment into three ranges: A (<2000 euros), B (>2000 euros) and C (>30,000 euros).

A quantitative calculation allows us to make a predictive analysis for use before making the investment or to analyze its profitability once it has been implemented. As a generic indicator, an innovation formula may be employed by dividing the share of innovation revenue by the total turnover multiplied by one hundred.

More specifically, we perform an analysis that considers the ratio between net revenues and innovation costs (ROI); the investment recovery period (IRP), i.e., the time required to recover the capital invested; and the cost reduction or savings resulting from innovation (RAC).

## QUALITATIVE ANALYSIS: INDIRECT BENEFITS AND VALUE

The innovation process is associated with an intangible effect with indirect benefits that, although more complex, must also be measured. To this end, one of the tools used is measurement through patient satisfaction (PSS).

In that specific section (dimension: structure) we can ask the patient for a numerical evaluation in reference to the specific innovation that we have implemented. Using a Likert-type scale, we can obtain information on value from the patient's or team's perspective (CSS).

### RECAP

>>>> **Idea 1** Innovating is changing our way of thinking and doing.

>>>> **Idea 2** Innovation is not limited to the incorporation of new technologies.

>>>> **Idea 3** Innovation adds value and makes us more competitive.

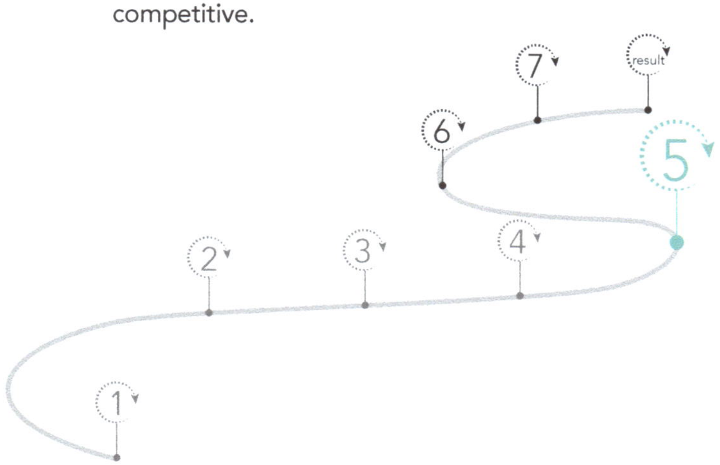

# EXCELLENCE

## A new way of understanding dentistry

Listen to *Alone in Kyoto*, by Air

36 min

Reading time: 36 minutes

1 2 3 4 5 6 7 result

Reading time: 2 min

# Excellence is in everything you do

*I learned the meaning of perfectionism by making sushi. Even before I had been to Japan, I felt a passion for its culture.*

*A Japanese dentist whom I deeply admired and whom I met in the United States told me that the best way to perfect advanced dental esthetic techniques was to learn* shodō *(Japanese calligraphy).*

*As a good disciple, there I was, in a small town near Kyoto, not quite sure what I was doing there, but delighted to have the opportunity to visit those landscapes and temples I had read so much about.*

*Aiko was a master craftsman and calligrapher from whom I learned to remain silent for hours and I confirmed that Japanese calligraphy is an extremely complex art!*

*His son, Haku, had a small* ryokan *(traditional lodging) in which he prepared dinner every night. Because of my passion for* sushi *and his great hospitality, he offered to help me after my classes. It was a unique opportunity to deepen my understanding of this culinary art. Every night I was fascinated to see how Haku and his lady prepared each piece, with attention to every detail, taking their time.*

*From those wonderful days I spent with this family, I especially remember our dinner conversations. Although the couple did not speak very fluent English, the talks were very enriching and a lot of fun. I especially remember one phrase that Haku said to me the night before I returned to Spain, when I asked him about the secret to making good sushi:*

*"Dear Laura, this is a matter of knowledge, technique and passion."*

# Excellence is an attitude

Reading time: 2 min

*"Excellence is not a destination, it is a way of traveling."*
*M_CONCEPT*

One of the objectives to which you should aspire as a professional is to be excellent in your daily practice, i.e., to commit yourself to a model based on quality care and continuous improvement.

Implementing a model of excellence requires a dentist to acquire new knowledge and skills. Working with this approach involves approaching each day as a challenge, an opportunity to correct mistakes and learn.

A dental practice that is committed to excellence exceeds the expectations of its patients, positions itself as a leader in the sector and achieves high profitability.

Good practice is not enough to achieve professional excellence. Professionals who achieve excellence are those who, in addition to offering technical excellence, manage to develop a series of competencies that allow them to effectively manage all the processes that occur in their dental practice.

*"We are what we repeatedly do. Excellence, then, is not an act, but a habit."*
*Aristotle*

Business excellence is the sum of outstanding performance in your daily practice and the way you manage your clinic to achieve specific results. This requires constant planning and supervision. It is not a one-time action, but a continuous cycle that is implemented and allows us to understand the level of performance and establish priorities for improvement.

In M_CONCEPT we have designed a management model oriented to dental practices that meets previously set quality standards in order to ensure predictable results.

Reading time: 6 min

# The quality formula

Health services can only have one level of quality: the highest. Quality is a concept that, *a priori*, may seem intangible, utopian or unattainable. In this section we will prove that quality of care can be measured and that this will be the path that will bring us closer to professional excellence.

For years, it has been identified that quality of care is of great value in organizations that provide services, such as dental practices. This is achieved with a strategy based on the definition, development and evaluation of processes to obtain results that ensure quality standards and perform periodic modifications. Thus, improvement is uninterrupted.

From this perspective, we can identify technical quality and functional quality. Technical quality is that which refers to health professionals, while functional quality is that which is perceived by the user or patient, both in terms of the final result of the service and its development.

At M_CONCEPT we will approach quality of care from an internal and external perspective, i.e. the final impact on the patient, so we will regularly analyze the quality perceived by the patient and the possibilities for improving the service they receive.

Due to factors such as intangibility, lack of knowledge of specific techniques, diagnostic criteria, etc., patients are often unable to accurately assess the technical quality of dental service, so functional quality is often the main determinant identified through their perception.

Therefore, a patient-oriented approach and the analysis of patient satisfaction is essential for patient attraction (potential patient) or patient loyalty (current patient).

To achieve this objective, it is necessary to understand the needs of users and to know what brings them value, i.e. what is really important to them.

Although there are multiple definitions of quality, in dentistry and in the model we will use as a basis, it is defined as "meeting or exceeding patient expectations in a rational manner." According to the UNE (A Spanish Standard]) EN-ISO 9000:2015 definition, satisfaction is the "customer's perception of the degree to which their expectations have been met."

It is important to know that even when the requirements have been agreed upon with the patient and met, high satisfaction is not assured. Therefore, it is necessary to go a step further and not limit ourselves to a minimum quality standard.

Clinics that achieve a high degree of patient satisfaction are those that understand and respond to their patients' needs and exceed their expectations.

This is why it is so important to measure this quality, a function that not only makes it possible to establish clear objectives, identify problems and compare the situation before and after the changes, but also provides the degree of patient satisfaction. This is quantified by analyzing the difference between their expectations (what they expect from the service) and their perceptions (what they perceive of the service provided).

Quality formula:
Quality = expectations - perceptions

The difference between perception and expectation will indicate quality deficits when the expectation score exceeds the perception score.

If perception exceeds expectation, it will imply a high perceived quality of service, and this will translate into high satisfaction with the service. If, on the other hand, perceptions are lower than expectations, the result will be patient dissatisfaction.

$$P > E = \text{SATISFACTION}$$
$$P < E = \text{DISSATISFACTION}$$

Another way of putting it:

Patient satisfaction is a measure of how a dental practice's overall care performs in relation to a set of expectations. Patient satisfaction is generated when the patient's perception of the service is equal to or greater than the quality they expected from it, that is to say:

| Satisfaction formula:<br>Patient satisfaction = expected quality - perceived quality |
|---|

The quality expected by patients is based on aspects as diverse as: their current needs, previous experiences or information received from acquaintances, among others.

Expectations play a fundamental role, since whether the patient is disappointed or surprised upon contacting the clinic depends to a large extent on these expectations.

DOWNLOAD

Template 28: *Quality-satisfaction formula*

Reading time: 6 min

# Patient journey

Perceived quality is based on the patient's experience during each moment of interaction with the clinic, i.e., the moments of truth (MOT), which we have already discussed in Chapter II.

As you know, MOTs are the situations of contact or interaction between the patient and the clinic that shape the patient's experience. This experience will ultimately shape the patient's impression of the organization. These critical interactions can improve or worsen the patient experience and are directly related to patient perception.

In other words, patient satisfaction is an indicator summarizing the patient's experience (patient journey) through all MOTs. A single negative experience in one MOT can affect the overall experience, even if in all other aspects the performance was excellent.

Optimizing waiting room times, personalizing the service or providing an innovative, unexpected and memorable element will score positive points. These points are not always associated with large investments; sometimes, simply addressing a patient by name or remembering their child's soccer game can score positive points that add to the DCP. Thus, the way to influence patient satisfaction is to act on each of these components that define your service.

The DCP is made up of a multitude of very diverse factors, so for the patient satisfaction assessment to be useful, it must cover all its components. To do this, you must analyze their priorities, i.e., identify what is important to the patient with respect to the characteristics of your service.

Not all of these components are equally important in terms of satisfaction. Therefore, you must identify those aspects that have the greatest impact and relevance. Based on this analysis, you will obtain a hierarchy of improvement actions and distinctive factors that will boost your dental practice.

Resources are limited, so you must prioritize those actions with the greatest impact on patient satisfaction (valued by patients). To do so, you must carry out the patient satisfaction survey (PSS), divided into dimensions, from which you will obtain results that will later be analyzed by means of correlation models.

Using a graph divided into four sections, you will be able to see:

- Factors to maintain: of great importance, but low impact.
- Marginal factors: demands with low importance and low impact.
- Priority action areas: high importance and impact. These are the levers of satisfaction.
- Opportunities to surprise: low importance and high impact factors.

DOWNLOAD

Template 29: *Patient priorities*

Crossing the satisfaction results for the attributes with the importance of each attribute in relation to overall satisfaction, you will obtain another graph that guides you on the areas for improvement (left area) and the competitive advantages (right area) of the dental practice.

Based on this analysis you will be able to classify, according to the degree of satisfaction/loyalty:

- Committed patients: high satisfaction (≥9) and high loyalty (≥9).
- Hostage patients: low satisfaction (≤5) and high loyalty (≥9).
- Disappointed patients: low satisfaction (≤5) and low loyalty (≤5).
- Mercenary patients: high satisfaction (≥9) and low loyalty (≤5).

More than 90% of unsatisfied patients do not complain and do not repeat, so if you do not perform this assessment, you will not know the reasons why you have not achieved their satisfaction.

There are controllable and non-controllable factors (rules, regulations, etc.). Controllable factors are modifiable; on the other hand, non-controllable factors can be addressed. For example, you cannot change the legislation that regulates a sector, but you can inform, explain and communicate to your patients the implications it may have.

We will also address guaranteed elements and distinctive elements.

The first are those that refer to aspects that patients "take for granted," for example, that the dentist is legally licensed. If these are fulfilled, the patient will not be more satisfied, but, if these are not fulfilled, it will greatly impact their dissatisfaction, in addition to the relevant legal consequences.

On the other hand, distinctive aspects are those that allow you to win over the patient and differentiate yourself from the competition.

Your actions should be oriented, first and foremost, towards fulfilling the guaranteed elements. Subsequently, you should focus your efforts on distinctive elements.

Therefore, for the patient satisfaction assessment to be of value, it must consider their priorities and expectations, as well as optimal performance in outcomes related to their perception. Knowing patients better is the best strategy to create value. Analysis allows you to understand your problems, needs and expectations.

As we explained in Chapter II, to exceed patient expectations you must work on high quality values in order to obtain scores between 9 and 10 on the NPS scale.

SERVQUAL is a survey used to measure the quality of a service that considers the perceptions and expectations of a user.

In M_CONCEPT we have designed and adapted a patient satisfaction survey (PSS) based on the dimensions, priorities and peculiarities of dental care. The differences (or gaps) between perceptions and expectations must be analyzed and are the ones that will provide the proposals for improving the service offered.

Reading time: 12 min

# The quality method

There are different models for measuring the quality of organizations. These models can be adapted and applied in different areas.

Our ultimate goal is to work under the total quality philosophy, i.e., to focus on continuous improvement and not limit ourselves to error detection and resolution. This concept involves analyzing and comparing. To do so, we must have a method that allows us to measure and identify which elements are important based on facts and data (indicators), which we call *evidence*, based on previously established quality standards.

The M_CONCEPT model has been developed by the team at MBA dental® and represents an adaptation of quality care and professional excellence models to the dental sector. This model defines seven modules: strategy, differentiation, analysis, core, innovation, excellence and implementation.

This model proposes management with clinical application in which, through a series of tools and work protocols, the complete care process (before-during-after) is analyzed.

With the work developed over the years by the team of experts that comprise MBA dental® and the clinical expertise, we have selected the most relevant aspects of the main quality models and adapted them to create a unique model for the dental sector.

The concept of quality began in handicraft production and in industry and later moved into the service sector. With chain production, it became clear that the greater the conformity (quality) produced, the less waste and reprocessing, so that the cost of the production process and, therefore, of the product was reduced.

The concept of *total quality* (*Total Quality Management* —TQM—) was a management strategy developed by W. Edwards Deming in the Japanese industrial sector. It is oriented to the creation of quality in all the processes of an organization, considering the people who work in it. This author made great contributions such as the Deming cycle, also known as the PDCA cycle, which we will discuss in the following section.

The European Business Excellence Model, developed by the European Foundation for Quality Management (EFQM), defines the model as a tool for self-assessment and the determination of continuous improvement processes in both private and public business environments. The main concepts or characteristics that make up this model are: orientation towards the results; customer orientation; leadership and coherence; management by processes and facts; development and involvement of people; continuous learning process; innovation and improvement; development of alliances; and social responsibility of the organization.

The Malcolm Baldrige model or North American model of excellence is a tool for evaluation, improvement and planning. This model considers seven key points, which are used to evaluate the quality management system: leadership; strategic planning; customer and market orientation; information and analysis; human resource orientation; process management; and business results.

Given the complexity of some models, their unsuitability for a dental practice and the functional difficulty they would present, we have designed M_CONCEPT, a model adapted to the dental sector.

## HOW DO I GET STARTED?

Excellence is not improvised; it is organized through a method that allows planning and directing actions towards specific results.

A model of excellence allows any organization to perform a self-assessment or self-diagnosis through systematic reviews of its strategies and daily practices. In addition, it is important to foresee situations that may occur and design-simulate a plan that can be implemented quickly and efficiently.

Quality implies permanently improving the efficiency of the clinic and its activities with a permanent focus on patient's needs, as well as on their possible complaints or dissatisfaction.

The way you will measure the quality of care to achieve excellence will be through the implementation of basic standards of care and indicators and their subsequent verification (systematic evaluations).

## KMI FORMULA: KNOWLEDGE-METHOD-IMPLEMENTATION

To achieve professional excellence you must follow the KMI formula.

The acquisition of knowledge and the leader's and the team's specific preparation will be the first necessary step to understanding the management model and the concept of *care excellence*.

The next step will be to follow the guidelines in an orderly and systematic way to achieve results established via a method.

Finally, you will work on set-up and fine-tuning, i.e. the implementation of the management model, which will encompass the integration of all the areas covered.

## BUSINESS PROCESS MANAGEMENT (BPM)

*"If you can't describe what you are doing as a process, you don't know what you're doing."*

*Edwards Deming*

Since the publication of the ISO 9001:2000 quality management system, BPM has been incorporated into companies. Thus, a new approach was introduced, oriented toward the proper functioning of the system through processes, continuous improvement and customer satisfaction.

A business process management (BPM) system is characterized by the understanding, visibility and control of all processes by the team, in order to increase efficiency and patient satisfaction. With BPM, you will adopt a series of steps or actions that will modify your way of working, always focused on the patient (patient centric).

With a systematized care process, all team members will act in the same direction. This orientation will allow you to optimize processes, improve efficiency, facilitate decision-making and, ultimately, be more competitive.

We are going to define three important concepts in our model, which are sometimes confused:

- Process: set of interrelated activities and resources that transform input elements into output elements, providing added value for the patient.
- Procedure: one which explains in detail how to develop the process.
- Protocol: step-by-step description of all the procedures of each process that takes place in the dental practice, with no possibility for modification.

Depending on their purpose, processes are classified as strategic, operational or key, support and measurement.

- Strategic processes: define and control the goals of the dental practice, its policy and strategy. They are directly related to the mission/vision. They are carried out by the management or leader, but involve the team as a whole.

  Examples: strategic planning, description of the dental practice's mission and vision, design of tactics, internal/external communication...

- Operational or key processes: these enable the service provided to the patient to be generated, and therefore have a direct impact on the patient's final satisfaction. The management of operational processes has special consideration, given their importance, so they should be improved as a matter of priority and urgency, since they condition the success of the dental practice. They are carried out by all team members.

  Examples: patient care, satisfaction, loyalty...

- Support processes: these include the activities necessary for the correct functioning of operational processes. They are also called auxiliary processes.

  Examples: spare parts for consumables, computer software maintenance, supplier contributions, maintenance, team training...

- Performance measurement processes: are associated with control of compliance with requirements, detection of errors or deviations in the strategy/results.

  Examples: KPI analysis, OKR…

This model requires an initial investment of time, but, once implemented, it will be the structure that allows you to optimize your daily practice.

At this point we introduce the *Lean* methodology, an innovative way of managing processes aimed at eliminating non-value-added activities in order to provide a higher quality service and improve the patient experience. In other words, in efficient dentistry, the aim is to optimize both production and management processes, using fewer resources and providing more value.

M_CONCEPT is a dynamic and flexible model that can be adapted to the needs of each moment of the dental practice; for example, if it is a newly opened clinic, if you are implementing new technologies, if it is a mature clinic that requires renovation, new processes…

Processes should be identified and described prior to incorporation. Once you understand the procedure, it will be very easy for all team members to perform and execute. The implementation of new processes without incorporating them into this system will lead to disorganization and disruption of the model. All the information will be integrated into a process map, which will allow you to have a comprehensive view of what happens in your clinic in a simple and graphical way.

## THE GOLDEN TRIANGLE: INTERNAL AND EXTERNAL ANALYSIS

The comprehensive analysis of your clinic will be divided into internal and external. This is what is called the Golden Triangle, since your model of excellence will be based on these three vertices.

Therefore, you must measure quality through patient satisfaction (external analysis, PSS), team satisfaction (internal analysis, CSS) and performance, i.e. the degree to which the objectives set are met efficiently (internal analysis, KPIs).

Reading time: 8 min

# Continuous improvement cycle

*"Insanity is doing the same thing, over and over again, but expecting different results."*
*Albert Einstein*

Willingness and ability to adapt to patients' needs are the conceptual bases from which continuous improvement becomes a work style.

The circle of continuous improvement (Deming's circle) is the basis of any quality system and makes it possible to address all types of activities.

The analysis you are about to perform identifies the service attributes most relevant to patients, as well as areas for improvement. Therefore, once the weaknesses have been established based on the opinion and perspective of the patients along with the work team, it is time to start a continuous improvement plan. Based on these criteria, you will focus on priority actions for improvement.

The management process in any organization should be structured into four types of actions, which are usually represented by the continuous improvement cycle (P-D-C-A). This cycle makes it possible to achieve systematically established results and obtain reliable information for decision-making.

- *Plan*: in this phase, the objectives are established after determining the current situation, making a diagnosis and defining the problems or areas for improvement, prioritized in order of importance. The methodology is also developed and systematic measurement is planned.
- *Do*: in this phase, the work is performed and measurements are taken. It is important to establish control mechanisms to analyze progress or correct errors.
- *Check*: is the evaluation phase, in which the results of the actions and measurements are checked, as well as deviations from the established objectives.

- *Act*: In this phase, corrective actions are applied and the necessary quality improvements are established to increase the satisfaction of patients and the work team.

If results have been achieved, procedures should be standardized and systematized to ensure they are maintained.

Some of the benefits resulting from proper process improvement are:

- Resource optimization.
- Increased efficiency and performance.
- Increased productivity.
- Error prevention.
- Systematic and integral vision of the DCP.

This implementation can be carried out gradually, i.e., through continuous improvement; or by means of so-called reengineering, which is implemented in a short period of time, thus obtaining a radical change in the process without maintaining the existing one.

## BENEFITS OF WORKING WITH AN EXCELLENCE-BASED APPROACH

Excellent organizations are extremely productive and highly profitable.

This model will give you greater sensitivity to detect opportunities for improvement. Process efficiency will translate into improved people performance.

Quality of care is perceived and valued by patients and the work team, so it will be a differentiating factor that will increase competitiveness and improve the positioning of your dental practice.

*"Give them quality. That is the best kind of advertising."*
*Milton Hershey*

In addition, the internal analysis includes performance and the achievement of objectives, which closes the Golden Triangle of the M_CONCEPT model. Therefore, you produce benefits for your patients and your staff and improve your clinic's bottom line.

## RECAP

>>>> **Idea 1** Quality is measured and continuously improved.

>>>> **Idea 2** Excellence can only be achieved with an integral and permanent method.

>>>> **Idea 3** The Golden Triangle combines the three pillars of success of M_CONCEPT.

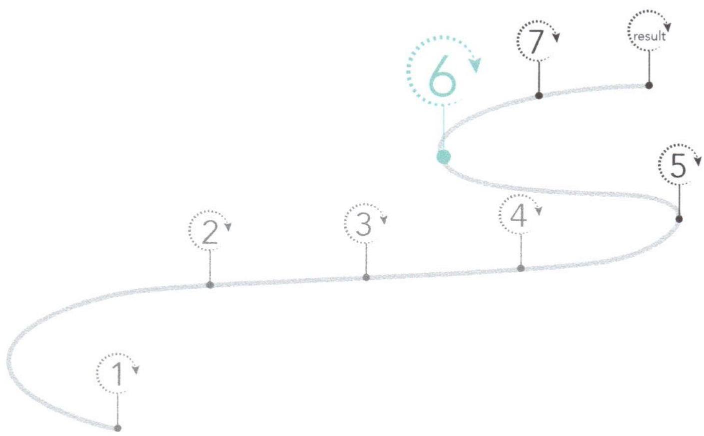

# IMPLEMENTATION

**It's time to take action**

Listen to *Right here, right now*, by Fatboy Slim

Reading time: 40 minutes

M

the

Reading time: 2 min

# The time is now

*During dinner with a professor at MIT (Massachusetts Institute of Technology), I had a conversation that would mark the following years of my teaching career:*

*Professor: Laura, I think you should launch that MBA project you designed for dentists and not put it off any longer.*

*Laura: I'm not sure, I've given it a lot of thought and the management model provides solutions, it's comprehensive and practical, but do you think a dentist is going to undergo training on this subject?*

*Professor: That's what you thought a few years ago, right? If a colleague proposed teaching you something you have never been taught that would change the way you approach dentistry, what would you say, would you be interested?*

*That knowledge is only useful if you share it. If you help other professionals improve their performance. That is the value of the hours you have dedicated to M_CONCEPT and the experiences that have led you here.*

*By this I do not mean that it will be easy; like anything new, you will have to put a lot of effort into making it known, into showing its importance and the impact it will have on dental practices. Do you think it is worth it?*

*The execution of a project is what brings value and produces results. Arnold Glasow said that an idea which is not linked to action will never be bigger than the brain cell it occupies.*

*If it is not a vital obligation, it will never be the time. For a great idea, for a great project…, the time is always now.*

*Find the right partners, test the model and launch it.*

# Integration of the M_CONCEPT model in the dental practice

Reading time: 2 min

*"The great aim of education is not knowledge but action."*
*Herbert Spencer*

As Albert-László Barabási pointed out in his formula for success, "as we advance in our careers, we become better at translating our ideas into high-impact outcomes."

To achieve excellence you must have a management model that ensures optimal organization, efficient use of resources and high staff and patient satisfaction.

You already have the knowledge and the method; now it is time to act, to put into practice everything you have been learning to get results in your dental practice. One of the main problems in any change process is not knowing where to start.

At this point you may find yourself in one of two situations:

1. Implementing nothing, i.e., continuing with the way things are and, therefore, getting the same results.
2. Starting to incorporate progressive changes that will boost your dental practice.

If you find yourself in the second scenario and you have really considered the entire contents of this book, you may feel so-called *analysis paralysis*. Therefore, we explain step by step how to perform the first actions.

*"The only thing worse than starting something and failing is not starting something."*
*Seth Godin*

Reading time: 14 min

# KMI Formula

To take these first steps we will follow the KMI formula: knowledge-method-implementation.

Before implementing, you should obtain information about the DCP and everything that happens in your dental practice. Thus, the first step is to understand and define the care process (DCP), since the improvement of care is achieved by understanding and analyzing the care process in a comprehensive manner.

Processes constitute what is done and how it is done. If processes are planned, improved and controlled, the organizational capacity and performance of your clinic will increase.

## Pre-during-post

Remember that dental care begins before your patient has visited the clinic, even before the first call for an appointment.

During the workflow you must control all factors according to the three dimensions described: people-processes-structure. Therefore, you must define all the processes that are part of the workflow and assign them functions and timing.

Processes should always be oriented, in function of the value chain, towards the objectives defined at all levels, so that they are aligned with the organizational vision of the dental practice. This is a strategic task to which you should dedicate time, because it will be the basis on which you will perform the daily activities of your clinic.

Next, you will need to implement the SASO method:

- S: systematization
- A: analysis
- S: stabilization-standardization
- O: optimization

## PHASE 1: SYSTEMATIZATION

*"Success is not only achieved through special qualities. It is above all a work of constancy, method and organization."*
*J. P. Sergent*

## WORKFLOW DESIGN: PROCESS MAP AND KPIs

Defining a coherent process structure, that represents the dental practice functioning, is the first step in understanding and organizing the care process.

All the activities carried out in the dental practice must be linked to each other and oriented towards offering value to the patient. This perspective will adapt to the needs and expectations of patients and improve the performance of the clinic.

From now on, you must understand the care process as a system made up of inputs that are transformed into a result or outputs.

Systematization is achieved through Business Process Management (BPM). Implementing BPM involves prior planning and the participation of all the people who are part of the team.

The resources you have are limited, so they must be organized and streamlined. Therefore, the more systematized your workflow is, the more optimized it will become.

Although the dental practice works with people, it is possible to automate certain processes to minimize variability and avoid errors. The key point is that before automating any process, it must first be identified, described and improved.

The graphical, orderly and sequential representation of all activities or groups of activities is called the *process map*. This diagram provides a clear view of the interactions that add value to the service received by the patient.

Therefore, the first thing you should do is to analyze and describe the DCP to understand the processes, model and optimize them, and then implement a system of protocols and automatization.

Each process will have the following data: process name and code, protocol, person in charge, execution time, priority assignment and method of evaluation.

The next step, after describing the processes and designing the process map, will focus on selecting the appropriate metrics (KPIs) to evaluate each process.

In summary:

1. Defining the processes and sub-processes of the workflow (pre-during-post).
2. Design the process map: relationships between the different processes.
3. Select metrics for evaluation.

# PHASE 2: ANALYSIS

## SITUATION DIAGNOSIS

In this phase, processes are followed up on and monitored to analyze results. During evaluation, corrective actions will be taken in the event of deviations or errors.

You must set measurable objectives that ensure everyone involved is working to achieve results. To do so, you will apply the OKR (Objectives and Key Results) method, which will allow you to efficiently achieve strategic goals. This system is used by companies such as Google, Twitter and Oracle, among others.

The method you use must meet the following requirements:

- Simple: to be implemented, it must be simple and easy to integrate into daily practice.
- Measurable: to have objective and comparable information, you must have a measurable system.
- Deadlines: results should have completion deadlines; this will maintain the team's focus and motivation.
- Accepted: the results achieved must be known, understood and approved by the work team.
- Flexible: this system must adapt to the needs of each moment and, therefore, be subject to modifications and redefined when appropriate.

Therefore, the design of the processes, the objectives and the results obtained must be aligned with our strategy.

The frequency at which the objectives are measured can be monthly, quarterly or annually. Metrics will be obtained from the *Golden Triangle*:

Internal analysis-KPIs: measurement of the clinic's performance through KPIs.

Internal analysis - satisfaction of the work team: measurement of the results obtained in the CSS (total average of the results obtained).

These surveys should be completed on a regular basis by all team members. The total average is obtained by taking the sum of the scores of all the items and dividing this by the total number of items. The overall results (≥8) are then analyzed and their continuity (three consecutive results) is established.

External analysis-patient satisfaction: results obtained through the PSS.

In order to monitor OKRs on a weekly basis, the P3 (progress, plans and problems) report should be prepared:

- Progress: what have you done this week to achieve the OKRs?
- Plans: what do you plan to do next week to help you achieve the OKRs?
- Problems: what problems, obstacles or delays have you identified that prevent or delay the achievement of the OKRs?

Analysis of results

In this second phase of the analysis you should focus on error detection and the continuous improvement cycle. The improvement phase aims to reduce the margins of variability within the process or to improve its levels of effectiveness and efficiency.

## PHASE 3: STABILIZATION-STANDARDIZATION

Stabilization is the phase in which previously established values have been reached consecutively over a period of time. The results measured both internally and externally mark the baseline or minimum level at which standardization can begin.

Standardization is the procedure by which processes are adjusted and adapted to a standard, i.e., to a model that is considered a reference.

Internal analysis:

- Performance: values equal to or greater than 80% must be obtained according to the KPIs for three consecutive months.
- Satisfaction of the work team: average results must be equal to or greater than 8 according to the numerical scale ($\bar{x} \geq 8$) for three consecutive evaluations.

External analysis:

- Patient satisfaction: values between 9 and 10 should be obtained ($\bar{x} \geq 9$), according to the NPS scale (Net Promoter Score) for three consecutive evaluations.

When you record the values indicated on the three vertices of the Golden Triangle you will be able to ensure that implementation is obtaining positive results and, therefore, proceed to standardization.

## PHASE 4: OPTIMIZATION

According to the Spanish Royal Academy (Real Academia Española), *optimizing* means "to find the best way to perform an activity." This concept, applied to the business environment, implies the need to plan and reorganize the resources available in the company in order to achieve the established objectives in the most efficient way possible, reducing costs and increasing profits.

In the final phase of implementation, once stabilization and standardization have been completed, the optimization process begins; i.e., efficiently obtaining the best result, using the least amount of resources. For this, the implementation of the M_CONCEPT model will allow you to progressively optimize time, people and material resources in each process.

Working with process-based management entails dedicating the right amount of time necessary to perform tasks and activities correctly from the outset, associating them with the person or persons responsible and with the necessary resources. In this sense, you will enter the continuous improvement cycle, so you will always be working in an optimal model with proposals for improvement.

For your dental practice to grow exponentially, all phases must be executed successfully.

DOWNLOAD

Template 30:
*Standardization-optimization*

# Act: action produces results

Reading time: 10 min

## DIRFT *MODE*

At M_CONCEPT we have incorporated part of the DIRFT philosophy (doing it right the first time), carried out by *Lean Manufacturing* (Lean Startup method: making the most of resources) and developed by Philip Crosby, which was based on the importance of doing things right from the start and his 14 steps to achieve it.

DOWNLOAD

Template 31: *Phil Crosby's 14 steps - quality (adapted)*

## ZERO-DEFECT DAY

Zero-defect day will be planned once you have passed the organization, data collection, initial implementation and analysis of previous results phases, in order to move on to the standardization of all processes.

To do this, you will need to set a specific day on which you will start with the goal of zero defects. In this case, you will work with a pre-established schedule and objectives to be achieved. You will follow the established phases and use the necessary tools for effective implementation. During start-up you must synchronize activities with respect to the three dimensions: people-processes-structure (PPS), in order to achieve optimization of the DCP.

If any of the phases have not been carried out successfully, you will not be able to proceed to zero-defect day. To do this, you must "roll" the system you have implemented by putting into practice the method explained. Before setting this day, organize a team meeting and make sure that everyone is informed of and agrees upon the starting day.

## DECISION-MAKING

In a company, decisions are made on a daily basis, both at a strategic and at a tactical or operational level. When making decisions, all information and alternatives must be analyzed logically and rationally, identifying potential problems or opportunities.

Information is the beginning and the end of the cycle, since the results and impact of each decision made will always be evaluated. Intuition or decision making based on other clinics or professionals carries a poor prognosis for the viability of your clinic.

Analysis is the basis for guiding decisions in a predictable manner.

## INFORMATION-DECISION-ACTION

As indicated at the beginning of the book, this model should help you organize and plan your clinical practice towards a focus on excellence and assist you in making decisions based on previously analyzed objective parameters.

The decision model must be aligned with the strategy you have set and oriented towards the objectives. The success of your dental practice depends on the number of good decisions you make.

When the action criteria are defined, it is easier to know how to handle daily and extraordinary decisions. In this philosophy, quality governs the decisions and activities of each and every member of the work team.

## BARRIERS TO IMPLEMENTATION

- Cognitive barriers: change and transformation initiatives can only be developed based on the integration of new knowledge. To this end, this book will serve as an introduction to the concepts you need to learn in order to incorporate a new management model into your dental practice.
- Resource barriers: the resources available to you may be material or human. You must also consider your most valuable resource: time. Implementing changes involves an initial investment of all of these. If implementation is done correctly, you will optimize these resources and even increase their value.
- Motivational barriers: moving from a theoretical model to a practical model is complex. One of the key factors is motivation, both your team's and your own as a leader. The best way to motivate your work team is to convey to them the importance of doing a good job and the benefits it will bring to the daily operation of the dental practice. To this end, it is essential to have their input and *feedback*, as this will lead to greater involvement.

Excellence is achieved with your work team (core).

A prerequisite for achieving objectives is a motivated, involved and committed team. Commitment to training and the professional and personal development of the team must be a fundamental pillar.

The satisfaction of all the people who are part of the clinic is the key to achieving the objectives. Their contributions to the improvement process should be valued and integrated into the implementation process.

In addition, working efficiently brings great benefits to the work environment, and this translates into the quality of care received by the patient.

## MYTHS

It is often thought that professional excellence entails a greater dedication of time, which is erroneous. It's not about quantity; it's about how things are done. Getting daily activities right from the start means effectiveness and the optimization of time and resources.

Another aspect that is often related to these models is that of work team control or dissatisfaction. Indeed, in a well-organized model, staff will have greater autonomy as they will have a perfect understanding of their roles. This will also allow processes to be carried out correctly, minimizing errors, which translates into less frustration and a reduction in the number of conflicts.

To get the most out of your team and optimize your time, you must delegate. To do this, the team must be trained and have clear guidelines.

Preparing for any possible scenario is what will make your dental practice more competitive and agile, and therefore more resilient to adverse situations.

## RESULTS

### EXCEEDING EXPECTATIONS

When you achieve stability in the processes that are part of your clinic's DCP, you will be at the right moment of maturity necessary to focus on further improvement. This consists of exceeding the quality expected by the patients and the team, which will be obtained from the information gathered in the internal and external analysis of the model.

The patient-person analysis will provide you with information to perfectly understand your target audience, offer the service they expect and exceed their expectations, always based on a high quality care process.

### FLEXIBILITY

As we have mentioned in previous sections, you already have tools that, together with the knowledge you have acquired, can be adapted to your needs.

These tools are dynamic, since your dental practice will evolve and, therefore, they must be adjusted to each moment and objective.

For example, when you reach high levels of satisfaction and achievement of objectives, you can modify the dimensions analyzed to focus on specific aspects such as the smell of your clinic or other kinds of details you want to analyze (distinguishing factors).

Therefore, the most important thing is to understand this model and put it into practice, although always with defined objectives and consistent with your strategy. Our recommendation is to initially focus on the key processes that enable your clinic to operate at its best, and progressively move towards more specific aspects that will allow you to differentiate yourself.

## EFFICIENCY

Efficiency is a mindset and should become part of the culture of your clinical practice.

Effectiveness is the simple achievement of goals or objectives proposed by the organization, while efficiency means achieving those goals through optimal execution, whether by requiring less time, spending fewer resources or any other circumstance that results in cost savings for the clinic.

This model is based on efficient dentistry, with quality criteria.

1 2 3 4 5 6 7 result

Reading time: 4 min

# Tips for successful implementation

## RECOMMENDATIONS AND ADVICE

At this point, it is important for you to be aware of the factors that will impede the effectiveness of this method.

What doesn't work:

- Partially implementing the model: as we have explained throughout the book, management must take an integral approach; focusing only on a few areas will not translate into stable results.
- Procrastinating: delaying organization, documentation and implementation increases the chances that you will not execute this project.
- Not relying on the work team: this is a task for each and every one of the members who are part of the processes of your dental practice.
- Finding excuses: I don't have time, it's a hard task, I have to focus on other things…
- Hoping for quick implementation.

What works:

- Working on all areas of management from an integral approach.
- Taking action from the outset, with a defined timeline and a start date for implementation.
- Engaging, training and working as a team, assigning tasks and functions and counting on their involvement in the strategic process.
- Discipline, self-demand and desire to excel: must be consistent, especially in the initial stages.
- Organizing progressive implementation: requires prior preparation.

## CONCLUSIONS: TIPS TO TAKE HOME

To design a successful clinic, you have found that excellent clinical practice is not enough, due to factors such as intangibility (the patient does not see, does not understand the treatment) and perception (for the patient there are other important aspects besides the treatment).

Therefore, we summarize ten key ideas that we hope you will remember after reading this:

1. Managing your clinic is a must if you want to achieve clinical excellence.
2. Managing your clinic involves analyzing and acting in all areas in an optimal way: strategy, differentiation, analysis, *core*, innovation, excellence and implementation.
3. Addressing only one area will not have a final impact on the management model or, therefore, on the results you will obtain.
4. An excellent clinic is based on achieving objectives (performance), a motivated team and a satisfied patient (in objective values).
5. If you don't measure, you can't improve.
6. To achieve an optimal management model, it is necessary to acquire specific training will allow you to make decisions that minimize risk and increase opportunities (eliminating intuitive decisions).
7. The commitment and involvement of your work team will be essential in this process.
8. Implementing a continuous improvement cycle will allow you to advance and grow.
9. Excellence is only possible if you have a method that leads to results.
10. This is up to you.

Reading time: 8 min

# Final thoughts

## ATTITUDE

From now on you must be observant and committed to continuous improvement; this will allow you to offer the best service to your patients.

Empathy, both for people and their circumstances, is a fundamental aspect of this process. A positive and optimistic attitude will help you motivate and transmit your work philosophy to the team, and this will be received by the patient.

You must also be self-critical and understand mistakes as opportunities for improvement. This is a fundamental aspect that you must accept before starting improvement actions.

## TEAMWORK

Your work perspective should always be based on teamwork. Each and every member must be committed and be part of this process.

Having different points of view, knowledge and experiences will enrich your knowledge of the care process.

## METHOD

To develop adequate management, you must have tools and be methodical; this way, you will minimize errors and improve compliance with the established objectives.

## MINDSET

The first step in establishing changes that produce results is to change your perspective, broaden knowledge and orient actions towards defined objectives.

At this point, I hope that the contents of this book have helped you to better understand the key aspects of providing excellent care.

Probably, if I had asked you about your objectives before reading this book, they would be related to increasing production, turnover... I hope you have understood that this will be the result of offering high quality service and optimizing your resources.

## TRAINING

*"Before everything else, getting ready is the secret of success."*
*Henry Ford*

Training in management is a must. Everything we have told you in this book is the beginning of your training.

From this moment on, we are sure that your interest will increase and we hope that learning in this exciting area will be one of your goals.

Your cognitive process (competence-awareness) has already begun.

## ACT: JUST IN TIME

Now is the time to start developing this method for three reasons:

1. The application of the knowledge you have acquired has greater impact now.
2. The motivation curve is always higher at the beginning.
3. Your mindset has already changed.

Remember that, in order for this reading to become the beginning of change, you must put into practice the knowledge you have acquired.

It's time to take action. To do so, we recommend that you follow the step-by-step implementation recommendations, make progress in the management of your daily practice and commit to taking your clinic to the next level.

Improvement is always possible.

*"Every person should undertake a major project at least once in their life. Now it's your turn. You must strive to create something that can benefit society."*

*Edwin Reingold*

Time is your greatest asset, and it is finite.

## RECAP

>>>> **Idea 1** Action delivers results.

>>>> **Idea 2** The SASO method coordinates sequences of actions.

>>>> **Idea 3** Efficiency simplifies and optimizes.

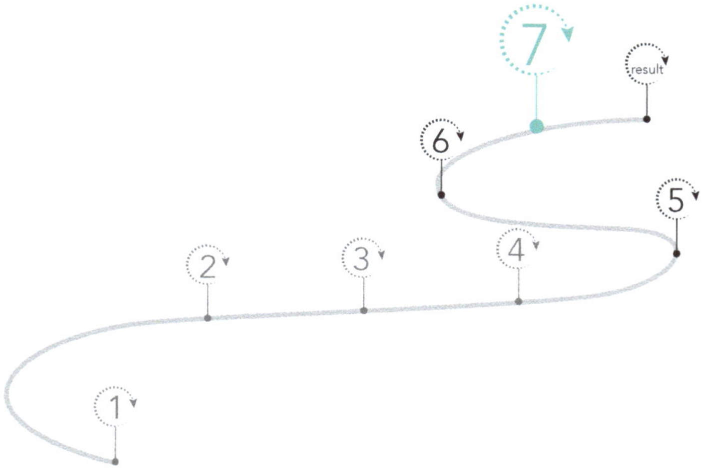

Reading time: 4 min

# BONUS TRACK

## The practice of the future

A question I am frequently asked is: *What do you think the "ideal practice" should look like?*

Businesses evolve at the same pace as society; therefore, a dental practice must be open to needs, changes and trends.

Most people who know my background expect an answer geared towards artificial intelligence (AI) or the incorporation of a new business model.

Successful companies are those that improve, change and impact people's lives. I think the dental practices that stand the test of time are those that are based on defined values. Although there are different approaches, factors such as ethics, responsibility and commitment to patient health are inherent to this profession. When your profession combines vocation, passion, dedication and devotion, success comes by itself.

Technology is a means to ease this process, but it is not the key should it be included as the only factor. As you have read in this book, innovation is more than just implementing technology in a dental practice.

The common factor among successful companies, in any sector, is innovation. Beyond the incorporation of new technology in the dental practice, it is a philosophy, a way of working, an approach that is implemented in all the processes of the dental practice and that has a great impact on the three cornerstones that determine excellence: patients, the work team (core) and performance, the **Golden Triangle**.

It all starts with a change in perspective that allows you to broaden the way you orient your dentistry. This is probably the greatest contribution we hope to have offered you, because it all starts with a change in *mind-set* (the why). You will then look for the knowledge, the tools and the procedure (the how). This equation is initiated by the why.

We truly hope that through this reading a first reflection or thought has been provided; also that the contents will be of great assistance.

# CONNECTING THE DOTS

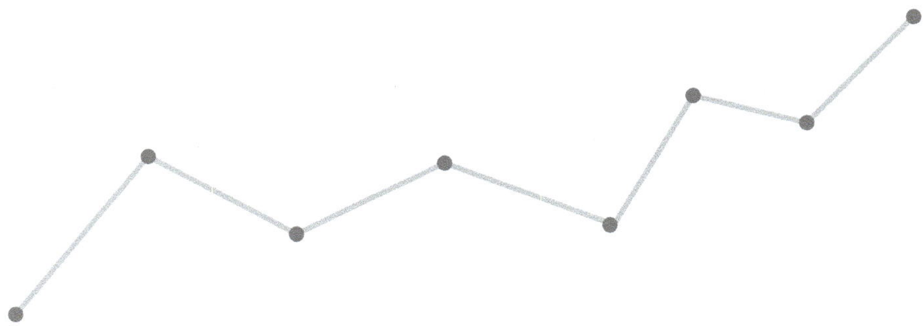

Reading time:
54 minutes

M

the book

Reading time: 6 min

# Dot 1. Set a goal you are passionate about and map out the route to achieve it

"The starting point of all achievement is desire," said Napoleon Hill. Indeed, performing an action implies wanting to do it.

*If I hadn't visited that dental practice and wanted to become a dentist, I probably wouldn't be here today.*

However, desire is not enough. Without planning, you are unlikely to succeed. Antoine de Saint-Exupéry reflected: "A goal without a plan is just a wish." I would add: "without a plan A and a plan B."

Both on a personal and professional level, to reach a goal you must make an initial time investment to plan how to achieve it. As Álex Rovira says, "good luck" has to be created. You have to work on the circumstances that will lead you to your goals. Defining each step towards that goal is the beginning (tactics). This action plan guides you and commits you to achieving it.

To this end, Jim Collins created a concept: BHAG®, acronym for *big, hairy, audacious, goal.* It was designed to define where you want to be in the next 10-30 years. Bill Gates laid out one of the most well-known BHAGs® in the world: "A computer on every desk, in every home."

## HOW DO YOU ACHIEVE YOUR GOALS?

Visualize your goal: mentally recreating the goal connects neurons, which reproduce it in the brain as if you were actually doing it. The subconscious is activated through your brain's reticular filter (RAS). When information passes through the RAS, it is converted into conscious thoughts and emotions.

Robert K. Merton said that our behavior is conditioned by what we anticipate will happen. That is why it is so important to project these objectives until they become reality. Keep your goals in mind, focus your subconscious and get closer to them.

Write down your goals: this is an explicit statement of your purpose and commits you to small actions that move you towards a result.

According to Dr. Gail Matthews, if you write down a goal, you increase the probability of achieving it by up to 42%.

Ashley Feinstein, in an article she wrote for Forbes, pointed out that writing down objectives gives us a reference and makes them more easily measurable.

Break it down: objectives can be set for the short, medium and long term.

*More than 15 years have passed from the day of my visit to that practice.*

It is important, therefore, when projecting into the long term, or if the final objective is a big challenge, to divide it into small goals.

Focus on the path, not the finish line: having a plan of action will allow you to determine a direction, focus your efforts and motivate yourself through small accomplishments (which raise dopamine levels!).

James Clear, author of *Atomic Habits*), suggests that we focus on the process, not the end result.

Scott Adams said that goals are the results you want to achieve and systems are the processes you follow to achieve those results. Focusing on those processes will help you progress.

Success lies in the path, not in the goal.

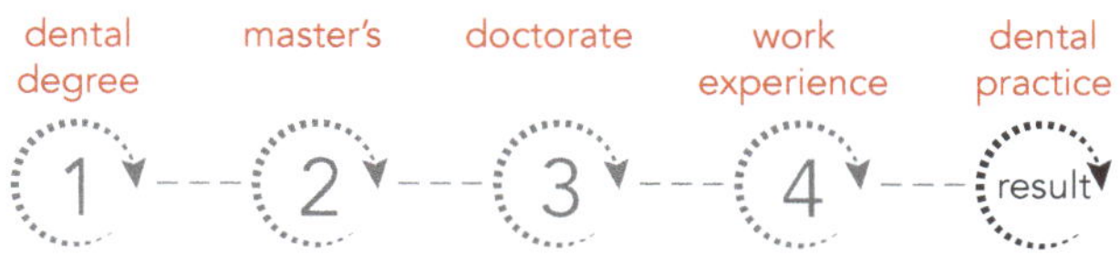
dental degree
master's
doctorate
work experience
dental practice
1
2
3
4
result

This objective can be shaped and adapted as you and your projects evolve.

*In this book you will see how, in my case, I adapted the objective of a dental practice to my own moment in life.*

Sometimes, our own daily rhythm takes us away from our goals. There is an expression that perfectly describes when we limit ourselves to working on a daily basis, without having a clear why and what for: *You're going nowhere fast.*

Don't let inertia move your goal, your practice or your objectives. Don't lose your vision, your purpose. Focus on maximizing opportunities and minimizing risks. This is all part of your strategy.

Stop; take the time to define what you really want and those actions that will mark your efforts in the coming years. In your practice, you must have a plan that allows you to achieve your vision, through your mission, in consistency with your values.

1 2 3 4 5 6 7 result

# Dot 2. Everything is communication

Reading time: 8 min

*Years ago I understood the importance of communication, as a holistic concept, for a dentist.*

Through communication, we present ourselves to a market and offer what we do best.

Through communication, strong teams and practices are created that are able to attract, engage and retain patients.

Through communication, we provide a unique experience that makes the difference.

*Since starting that class at the HSDM, I began to interpret all the information I was learning. That event inspired me about how to turn a care protocol into an unforgettable experience. Ever since then, I analyze every company I deal with, I learn from them.*

Do continuously learn about marketing: from now on, you must be fully aware and observe what the companies you like, of which you are a regular consumer, are doing. Assess what makes them different, how they do it and what impact those things have on you as a customer. Thinking like a consumer will help you to better understand your patient.

"Satisfaction guaranteed or your money back."

This business promise was launched by Montgomery Ward (founder of the first mail-order store) in 1875.

Commitment to customer satisfaction is a demanding promise. For this premise to be fulfilled, you must know them perfectly and, of course, be consistent with the message you are broadcasting. Their loyalty will depend on the degree to which you meet and exceed that business promise, i.e., their expectations.

From now on, you have a tool (PSS) that will allow you to measure the most important number for your practice: NPS.

Before communicating, you must define who you are, as a professional or as a dental practice. This is part of the strategy, so do not initiate communication until you have defined what you want to communicate. Consistency and the way you communicate are two key factors. Your dental practice must be aligned with the values it communicates. Your communication must also provide solutions to problems through your service.

Your personal brand is based on what makes you unique, what is known as your *uniqueness*. To start working, you must carry out an identification and definition process. Tom Peters, recognized as a guru of gurus by The Economist and Fortune, used to say that to define your *uniqueness* you must answer this question: *What makes you unique that no one else can offer?*

This process takes time and introspection, but the good news is that, even if you haven't defined it yet, you are already unique. Differentiation is the key to positioning.

> *"To get what only 1% of people get,*
> *just do what 99% of people don't."*
> *Anxo Pérez*

All this must be extrapolated to your practice: *What makes you different? How do you bring value to your patients?*

Your practice's communication is about conveying the benefits of your services effectively, so that your patients identify what you can do to meet their needs.

The mirror image of your practice, your communication, cannot be represented by an implant (you are not selling products). As you know, added value plays a key role. Spend time designing your value proposition.

Increase your patients' confidence: good communication will generate commitment from your potential and current patients. Ask them to share their experiences at the dental practice through reviews and comments.

A study published by Deloitte affirms that consumers trust *online* reviews as much as the opinions of family and friends. Adapt to these new forms of communication. Think like a customer. Have you ever chosen a hotel on Booking.com based on reviews and comments?

This data will have a great impact on your patients and will be useful for identifying the areas for improvement in the dental practice that are expressed in those comments.

Design WOW moments tailored to your patients: to connect with your patients you need sensations, experiences and emotions. Achieving an emotional bond with your current or potential patients, so that they feel the brand is their own and want to be part of it, will be the focus of new communication strategies.

Quality and price put you in the league; service distinction wins it. To do this, you must design an atmosphere that revolves around the sensory and emotional, i.e., that attracts the patient and allows them to enjoy the experience through the combination of more than one sense: multisensory.

To this you must add the surprise factor, which defines the experience. This will result in three key points:

1. That your patient comes back (loyalty).
2. That they communicate and share their positive experiences with their local environment (referrers).
3. That you leave the competition behind.

Don't forget about internal communication: usually, dental practices direct their efforts towards external communication; however, the most complex interactions occur with your team and are the most important. In this type of communication, aspects such as continuity, personal relationships and emotions make it more intense and complex.

Internal communication is not only about informing the team, but also about an evolution of the corporate culture that involves and builds the loyalty of the team *core* in all processes of the DCP. Controlling this communication will allow you to express yourself effectively at an external level. You must understand communication as a competence in which you must train and prepare yourself.

Dentists can learn to communicate better. Dental practices as well.

# Dot 3. The power of information

Reading time: 6 min

Data are the key elements for the development of your dental practice: without them, it will be difficult to correctly direct all efforts towards greater profitability.

*It was clear to that entrepreneur of a small coffee shop that knowing and measuring the needs of his customers was the key to growth. This allowed him not only to build loyalty, but also to design a formula to reproduce a business model.*

*"Get closer than ever to your customers. So close that you tell them what they need well before they realize it themselves."*
*Steve Jobs*

Niels Bohr said "An expert is a person who has made all the mistakes that can be made in a very narrow field."

The most frequent mistakes made by a dental practice are already defined. Your goal will be to prevent and anticipate them. However, as you know, in this model we are not satisfied with just doing things right. To this end, we will go one step further through a zero-defect system.

Your source of learning and improvement is centered on your patients, your team and all the objective data that define your daily practice.

*Every time I receive a satisfaction survey from a hotel, a flight or any other company, I not only take it, but I look at every item it reflects.*

All successful companies are *customer centric*: make your practice patient centric, get closer to the needs of your patient.

Focus on the patient, not the competition.

Numbers can be your best ally.

*The first time I met with my business manager I was aware that, although I was a dentist, I needed training in financial matters. I now know that in order to practice within a margin of safety, to grow and to ensure the viability of my companies, I must be prepared in this area.*

*A priori*, dealing with "numbers" does not usually appeal to us and, moreover, it is a complex subject. I assure you that, in order to meet your financial obligations and make decisions that allow you to enjoy your profession, you must be fully aware of your economic model. Financial training allows you to give your dental practice sustainability.

I think something that happens to most dentists is: "it works for me." You think you generate enough income to cover your needs. This attitude is comfortable and simple, but it puts you in a complicated situation if changes occur in the environment.

When you take a close look at the numbers, you become aware of unnecessary expenses, explore opportunities and visualize what you can optimize. Closing your eyes does not exempt you from your responsibility as an entrepreneur, so this analysis must be carried out, and the sooner the better.

> *"Reality is merely an illusion, albeit a very persistent one".*
> *Albert Einstein*

Being prepared will allow you to make decisions with calculated risk. This knowledge will be useful in your daily practice and also in the most adverse situations. It will also allow you to perfect your business model.

Jim Rohn said: "The key factor that will determine your financial future is not the economy; the key factor is your philosophy."

Financial intelligence is a skill related to our knowledge and view of money, which guides our decision making. Normally, if you are not in a finance or accounting-related profession, you do not usually acquire this type of knowledge. In the case of dentists, we are forced to do it when we start out.

Achieving stability and, better yet, financial freedom is something that can be achieved with the right knowledge. Financial freedom occurs when passive income covers all expenses.

The virtue of giving before receiving: something else I have learned from great entrepreneurs is that your company's profits are essential, but not the reason for its existence. You will only generate profit if you provide solutions, well-being, usefulness and value to other people.

*Brian Swann, my mentor at the Harvard School of Dental Medicine (HSDM), taught me that we dentists have a duty to serve and help our patients and society. It is our responsibility as health care providers. It really surprised me that one of the most elite universities in the world had programs that involved its students and taught them about the role of a dentist and their social commitment.*

It is essential to understand that money should be a means, not an end. Henry Ford said that a business that produces nothing but money is a poor business.

*A business guru from whom I have learned a lot told me that, in the new business paradigm, successful organizations will be those that work out of passion and service to others.*

You get back what you give: as an entrepreneur and as a dentist you must keep in mind your commitment to your patients. Your goal, therefore, is to perform an activity that brings meaning to your life and to the lives of others; to maximize service, not profit. Thus, income will be the consequence.

> The prosperity of your dental practice will be proportional to the solutions you provide to your patients in an excellent way.

Offering what you do best with will, vocation and passion will give solidity to your business project.

Reading time: 6 min

# Dot 4. The importance of people

Companies are made up of people: they are the most important asset you can have. Your goals will only be achieved with the help of others. Your time and knowledge are limited; there will come a time when you will have to delegate in order to grow. And, honestly, the trip is more enjoyable and enriching! The path of an entrepreneur is full of obstacles; careful selection of the people who will be at your side will be of utmost importance.

*The event that happened to me in England is very simple. Sometimes, turning points arise from everyday experiences. For me, being able to work with people from different cultures and with different outlooks on life was a great help in understanding the relationships within a work team.*

*Fortunately, being a worker and a leader gives you a very enriching two-way view.*

*Like many dentists, when I started my business project, I had no training in this area, which, in addition to my immaturity, caused me to make guidance mistakes over and over again with my work team.*

The "human equation" is not a mathematical formula. However, there are universal conditions that make people feel integrated, motivated and involved in a common objective.

The true meaning of leader: a concept that changed my understanding of leadership was that described by Jim Collins. According to this author, a level 5 leader is a person who combines extreme personal humility with a strong professional will. In other words, they prioritize what they can build, create and contribute according to their needs or personal ambition. These people are catalysts in the transition from good to excellent, which entails a very important process of maturity and personal development.

Good leaders empower others. The more you help others, the more they will want to help you. This creates a solid network of connections that will boost your career. You will be the inspiring example for your team, so leadership starts with you. Subsequently, there are three aspects that you must not forget (CTT): communicate, train and trust.

Encourage feedback from your team (*what?* and *why?*), make it easier for them to perform their tasks through training and means (*how?*) and, finally, delegate, give them autonomy to make them feel fulfilled with the work they perform in your dental practice.

> *"The best teamwork comes from men who are working independently toward one goal in unison."*
> *James Cash Penney*

Show availability to help them and reward them. Serotonin levels flow when they feel they are important and significant to the practice. Sometimes it's just a matter of recognizing what they are doing well. Value the contributions of each person who is part of your team.

The right *core* at the right time: in addition to the importance of leadership, choosing the right people at the right time is a condition for success. You and your team must have a shared vision and the same goals, and be honest about what that entails.

People have different ways of understanding work, effort and goals. The sooner you identify whether they are the right partner for you, the less frustration for both parties. Selecting this second family is very important. To build engaged and committed teams, you must ensure that they are aligned with you and your dental practice.

Your role, subsequently, will be to articulate to each person their specific role. Last but not least, you must keep these people close, i.e., build a lasting relationship.

The book *Good to Great* discusses three aspects to being thorough when making decisions about the team:

1. If you have doubts about someone, don't hire them, keep looking.

2. If you know you have to make a personnel change, do it.

3. Assign your best workers the best opportunities.

I know how hard it is to make decisions about the people in your practice. This is one of the most complex aspects. However, I firmly believe that training will help you understand, manage and make better decisions. Remember that your team will be what helps you achieve success or, conversely, helps the project fail.

The reason you get up every morning: when you feel good about your work, you face the challenges of each day with enthusiasm and creativity and you minimize or solve problems better, which, in turn, is related to productivity. Having a reason activates the ikigai (vital motivation) and mobilizes talent, passion, that which makes you get up every morning with enthusiasm.

A significant percentage of time in your life is spent working. Do you think it is relevant to feel good while doing it? The core and the work environment are largely responsible for this well-being. Take care of your team and your team will take care of you and your patients. Failure to do so will lead to a reduction in productivity, effort and motivation and, ultimately, the loss of talent in your dental practice. Empathy and active listening are the keys to improve these relationships.

*Today I can assure you that no business project I lead could have been a reality without the people who are part of them.*

## Dot 5. Innovation is progress

Reading time: 8 min

It's a matter of perspective. Lateral thinking seeks solutions to problems with different, unusual ideas, via which we find alternative solutions.

The key to innovating in your dental practice is to develop that kind of thinking and to listen to all ideas/suggestions/complaints from your team and from your patients, suppliers or collaborators.

*"Whatever made you successful in the past, won't in the future."*
*Lew Platt*

The environment you are and will be in for years to come is changing rapidly: what made a dental practice successful ten years ago is now obsolete. Therefore, you must look for new opportunities and stay ahead of the market. Getting out of your dental chair will help you see everything from a different, less biased perspective. Broadening your perspective will allow you to identify more opportunities.

With innovation, you can interact in a highly dynamic and competitive environment. Think of companies like Uber, Youtube, Airbnb, Netflix or Amazon, which emerged from the shortcomings and needs of each sector, even those undetected by users.

*In my case, working with a multidisciplinary approach and sharing my profession with experts from other areas has allowed me to have a more holistic and integral approach to dentistry. This perspective has had a great impact on my clinical practice.*

Staying one step ahead will always help you position yourself as an industry leader. Let's take a look at a real-life example of the decision-making tree when implementing innovation in the dental practice.

The trend in dentistry, as in other biomedical disciplines, focuses on the individualized diagnosis and treatment of our patients. When we consider the possibility of providing genetic analysis in the dental practice, we ask ourselves: *Is it consistent with my strategy? Does it bring value to my patients? Is it an improvement in my diagnostics and treatment? Is it a viable innovation?*

Before implementing innovation, we must answer these questions:

*Consistency with our strategy*

> *Our approach is multidisciplinary and holistic, i.e., we do not limit ourselves to the oral cavity, but understand health as an integral concept.*
>
> *Our work philosophy is based on minimally invasive dentistry (MID) applied to all areas (surgery, periodontics, orthodontics, endodontics...).*
>
> *DNA analysis provides us with information of great diagnostic value and is a painless test with no side effects.*
>
> *Our values include innovation and excellence; therefore, the incorporation of this test is aligned with what we believe and invest in.*
>
> *This test allows us to differentiate ourselves through a new service, with great therapeutic potential. We were the pioneers, the first and, therefore, the reference practice.*

*Value for patients and diagnostic-therapeutic improvement*

> *The most common oral pathologies have a genetic component that, until now, has been unknown or undiagnosed at a clinical level. Systemic pathologies have a direct relationship with oral and dental pathologies, and this relationship is bidirectional. With this test, we can determine the predisposition to tooth decay of a two-month-old baby who does not yet have teeth. We can diagnose the severity of periodontal disease or detect celiac disease before the patient has their first contact with gluten.*

*Can you imagine how this changes the treatment paradigm?*

> *Genetics is not preventive dentistry, but predictive. It allows us to detect pathologies even in subclinical stages, before they present clinical symptoms, and to establish a treatment plan in the early stages (early intervention). This has a great impact on the prognosis and evolution of a disease, which makes it a test with high diagnostic and therapeutic potential.*

*Feasibility of incorporation into daily practice*

> *The sample is taken from buccal mucosa or saliva, so it makes sense for this type of test to be performed in a dental practice. The test takes five minutes, its transport does not require special conditions (as in the case of blood samples) and the information (DNA, proteins, etc.) is the same as that found in blood.*
>
> *The learning curve is fast and equipment training can be completed in one weekend. Its integration into daily practice is similar to taking impressions and sending them to the laboratory. The cost is affordable and assumable by the dental practice and our patients.*
>
> *The reliability and safety of the test exceeds 98%. These are analyses based on scientific evidence that have been carried out in other fields for over ten years.*
>
> *The incorporation of this test increases our reputation, patient turnover and profitability (ROI).*

Analyzing the information, it presents advantages that are fully aligned with our dental practice and brings value through innovation. This has a great impact on the added value mentioned above.

Our practice differentiates itself by providing a new service. Therefore, this incorporation adds to our communication and positioning strategy. This also implies a new care protocol, which will be designed during the first appointment and will be part of the patient experience (viewing results in 3D).

As you can see, prior to the incorporation of any innovation, you must carry out an exhaustive analysis, both quantitative and qualitative. If it is not profitable, sustainable and communicable or does not add value, do not implement it, even if it is a novelty. If you incorporate it, you must periodically evaluate the investment and the return, not only in economic terms, but also in terms of satisfaction (patient-team) and care improvement.

Nearsightedness is solved by changing your perspective: when you are within the walls of your practice, you limit your vision and, therefore, your evolution.

Rowan Gibson said: "If you're a bank, you think like a bank. If you are a supermarket, you see the world as a supermarket." Therefore, if you are a dental practice, you will think like a dental practice. This is a mistake, since it is when the focus is changed that a differential value is really provided. If you follow the inertia of the industry and the competition, you will do the same thing and get less and less results.

Training in different areas, working with an interdisciplinary approach, learning from people who do something different from what you do...; in short, opening your field of action, being open to new ideas and eliminating barriers will help you reconfigure your practice.

If you change, everything changes: the essence of innovation is curiosity. A first step is to continually question what you are doing, check if you are doing it right and if you could do it better.

Charles Darwin understood that being inspired by error was the starting point for critical reasoning. In his theory of biological evolution by natural selection, he described the importance of species adapting to the environment for survival.

Something similar happens in the business environment. Companies that do not adapt to the environment disappear. It is mistakenly believed that it takes a lot of resources to innovate. The essence of innovation focuses on changing or expanding your way of thinking. Observing everything that happens around your practice, listening to the people around you and being attentive to changes will drive you to innovate.

Design a creative environment in which the contribution of each member of your team is recognized.

*"The illiterate of the 21st century, will not be those who cannot read and write, but those who cannot learn, unlearn and relearn."*
*Alvin Toffler*

In short, we propose that you think differently in order to do something different, something that adds value. Through this model, we help you and your dental practice become a dynamic, flexible and resilient company. It's just a matter of perspective.

# Dot 6. From good to excellent

Reading time: 6 min

The road to excellence is always under construction: it is an ongoing process. Once you have decided that you want to achieve it, you are always committed to improving. Excellence flows from the inside out. Excellence starts with you and, later, with your practice.

Unless your patients are 100% satisfied, you must improve and, even then, you will have to keep surprising them and adapting to their new needs, which requires constant review.

Importantly, excellence does not depend on the size or turnover of your practice. There are patterns of action that determine excellence and that, despite what you may think, are within the reach of any practice.

Knowledge is the first step towards excellence. The more ambitious the goal to which you aspire, the greater your preparation must be. Your chances of success will increase in proportion to your training. Undoubtedly, this is your best bet if your goal is to grow personally and professionally. I am a firm believer in this.

*I have invested many hours in my training in different subjects. I have completed master's degrees, I have read hundreds of books. I have attended and participated in conferences, courses and trainings. Every hour spent has brought me one step closer to my goal.*

*"Learning how to learn more effectively is life's most important skill."*

*Tony Buzan*

Never put a limit on knowledge. Never stop learning. Never stop renewing yourself.

*As Haku said, we can all be excellent; it's a matter of knowledge, technique and passion.*

Passion and vocation are the engines that drive us to continue to evolve: they are responsible for the hours we dedicate to this profession, for continuing our training, i.e., for the time and effort we invest in it.

Enjoying this "sacrifice" is fundamental. Loving what you do is an essential factor in this equation. T. D. Jakes said that if you cannot discover your purpose then, discover your passion, as it will lead you directly to your purpose.

Have you ever wondered why some people enjoy their profession? There are factors at work that trigger the release of neurotransmitters related to happiness. Performing an interesting treatment, achieving a challenge, designing a creative activity... brings satisfaction and rewards performance. When you feel motivated, dopamine levels rise and you become more productive, so your abilities are enhanced. When you get into this dynamic, you become nonconformist. If you do things right, you will want to do them even better. You will continually ask yourself how you can progress.

You can always move forward, the key lies in attitude: excellence is based on small daily efforts, on details that end up making a difference.

We have already mentioned the importance of attitude in this entrepreneurial process and how it can determine the success of any type of project, whether personal or professional. This can start with incorporating habits into your daily life: being on time, running an extra kilometer, not giving up a language course, quitting smoking... In other words, setting small demands that lead you to fulfill a purpose. Be an improved version of yourself every day. If, in addition, you incorporate healthy habits that help you improve your quality of life, the change will be substantial. Taking care of yourself inside and out will increase your performance.

Achieving excellence is as important as maintaining it. Therefore, you must be consistent and constant. This is when discipline comes into play, which will set the guidelines to lead you to success. This takes some initial effort, but I can assure you that the results will change your life.

Some tips that have helped me:

- Surround yourself with people who inspire you, who teach you.
- Be curious, observe, research and learn from everything, even outside the dental industry.
- Work on critical thinking.
- Eliminate everything irrelevant; concentrate your efforts, focus yourself.
- Make everything around you simple. Success is based on efficient simplicity.
- Anticipate the market, your competition, even your patient.
- Don't settle for essentials, work on distinguishing factors.

There is no single factor that will make your practice excellent, but rather the combination and sum of all of them. For this reason, we propose a multi-factor model, which must be approached comprehensively and simultaneously. With these ingredients for success, you will be the one designing the recipe.

Reading time: 8 min

# Dot 7. To act or to act

Vincent Van Gogh said: "What would life be if we had no courage to attempt anything?"

*It's been six years since the first edition of MBA dental® and more than ten since the inception of the design of M_CONCEPT. When this adventure began, I didn't imagine the scope it would have.*

*I can tell you about all the data we have collected over the last few years and that we analyze in each edition. Among those we highlight is our last teaching evaluation, in which we obtained (on a Likert scale 0-10) an average of 9.98 or a score of 10 from 98% of our students on the item "degree of recommendation."*

*I can also point out that we started with a small group and that we currently have students who travel from more than ten countries to study at MBA dental®. Or that thanks to all the students and practices that have bet on MBA dental®, we continue to improve, grow and perfect our teaching and clinical methodology.*

*But something difficult to explain is what has been created after those hours of class, after those master's moments, after those experiences that united us in each edition. I remember edition I with special affection and enthusiasm. They were our pioneer students, a very heterogeneous group with whom we connected from the beginning of the first session. We began to learn from them by receiving feedback on the implementation of M_CONCEPT and analyzing its clinical impact.*

*This has continued in each edition. Our students have not stopped surprising us and showing us that being excellent is an attitude; an attitude with which we must work every day to achieve excellence.*

*That was the beginning of a project that has exceeded all our expectations. We knew that at MBA dental® we were going to meet great professionals, but what we didn't know was what they were going to contribute to us inside and outside the classroom.*

*When I go back to that moment, when I was uncertain about whether or not to launch the first MBA for dentists based on M_CONCEPT, I thank all the professionals who were the driving force behind its inception.*

*The transition from certainty to uncertainty is always complicated. It is very common for us to wait for an opportunity to come along as an ideal moment, but, in reality, the circumstances for opportunity are created and depend on you. If you wait for that "ideal" moment, you will always have an excuse for not leaving your comfort zone, for not taking risks, for staying in your current situation.*

We are surrounded by opportunities, but sometimes we do not detect them or we simply have an excuse not to take the step.

Albert Camus said that he who lacks courage always finds a philosophy that justifies it. The crisis, the pandemic, saturation, intrusiveness, franchises, competition... Sound familiar?

The time is now. Action produces results.

*Let me tell you a brief anecdote. One of the projects we had been working on for months was based on an international multidisciplinary face-to-face training program centered around minimally invasive dentistry (MID), taught by leading educators from several countries.*

*To this we added a learning experience in a unique environment (see QR code) that would allow the learner to optimize their training in a different way.*

*With seven days left to launch the project and publish the annual course schedule, an unexpected situation not only changed the course of the project, but also of the world: a pandemic (SARS-CoV-2) occurred and the subsequent* lockdown.

WATCH

Video: *A paradise called Tarifa*

*This situation led to a serious health, social and economic crisis. As far as this project was concerned, after so many hours of dedication and excitement, it was a big blow to the team.*

*When we met it was the beginning of the pandemic, we did not yet know the scope and impact it would have. During that time of extreme uncertainty, we had two options: to lament, get frustrated and give up, or to find an opportunity, even in such an adverse scenario.*

*It was during those days that we realized dentists were spending more time training from home. It took weeks of working against the clock, re-adaptation, late nights…, but we finally managed to articulate a portfolio of courses with a 100% online modality and high quality content.*

*We had the teaching team, the content and the students; we just had to change the format (think differently, innovate…). We improved our audiovisual resources, invested in portable recording systems, learned all about the online modality and activated our imaginations, even providing students with at-home work kits.*

*SOHO Academy® was born in the midst of a crisis, and was the result of proposing new ideas and alternatives adapted to the opportunities arising from critical situations. That is one of the most important lessons I have learned in recent years: opportunities are created, not awaited.*

*Our vision at MBA dental® goes beyond being a master's degree. We truly believe in improving the lives of dentists through a management model that leads them to achieve their goals. Every minute we have dedicated to this model has exponentially multiplied everything we have received. That is the difference between being just another master's degree and having a vision that goes beyond the limits of teaching.*

*As in all projects, this is the beautiful part (and the one that will certainly stay with us), but there have also been moments of frustration. On this road we have encountered obstacles, people who have not believed in this project, criticism, plagiarism, exhausting work days…; but, in spite of this, all we can say is that it has been worth it.*

Fortunately, when you believe in a project, none of the above can stop it. You just have to be consistent and try again. All companies go through moments of crisis; excellent companies failed at some point, don't feel bad if it happens to you. The difference at this point will just be whether you get up, learn and continue or, on the contrary, give up.

### Don't do it, don't quit!

If Thomas Edison tried thousands of times without losing faith, then you, just because of an obstacle, are not going to be frustrated. Each obstacle will bring you closer to your final goal.

Do you believe in the impossible? Check out the incredible story of Dick Hoyt and his son Rick (Team Hoyt).

The capacity of human beings to overcome adverse situations is incredible. Transformative action drives us to achieve impossible goals.

*"Persistence is the virtue by which all other virtues bear fruit."*
*Arturo Graf*

All you need is perseverance, a strategy to guide you and to believe in what you do.

1 2 3 4 5 6 7 result

Reading time: 6 min

# Connecting the dots: the result

*"You can't connect the dots looking forward; you can only connect them looking backwards."*

*Steve Jobs*

Dreams are only fulfilled if your motivation and effort overcome your fears and obstacles. If you believe in your project, you consciously choose to shape it and make it a reality. From that moment on, your efforts are directed to fulfilling it.

A year ago I moved to a paradise called Tarifa. It is a corner in the province of Cádiz (Spain). It is the southernmost point of the Iberian Peninsula, dividing the Mediterranean Sea and the Atlantic Ocean. It is a unique place where the wind and waves converge on wild beaches, dunes and natural parks. This place is a dream come true for any surfing, windsurfing or kitesurfing lover. For me, it was that idyllic place you dream of living someday... maybe when I retire.

During that stop, after years of such intensive work, I reflected on what I really wanted. Challenges and dreams are there to be met; we just need to lay out the strategy to achieve them. In my case, I needed to open my mind, align the three circles (BHAG®) and have a method to help me achieve it.

This may seem a long way from what you've read so far, but you're sure to make sense of it if you connect the dots that lead to the result.

M_CONCEPT is more than a management model, it is a philosophy that marks your way of thinking and acting. It is a tool that guides you and helps you achieve your goals.

This gave rise to SOHO, a different way of understanding dentistry. SOHO dental® is a practice concept that we have been working on for the last few years that combines all the concepts of M_CONCEPT.

This dental practice is based on differentiation through excellence and innovation. It is M_CONCEPT applied 100%. The innovation is based on the management model; the patient experience and the treatments performed, under the philosophy of minimally invasive dentistry (MID). During its development, we compiled each step so that a dentist will know everything they need to analyze before starting a business project.

SOHO will be extrapolated to other cities, so that a dentist who wishes to understand it in depth and develop this business model will be supported by our team from inception to start-up.

We are betting on designer dentistry, a dentistry based on our values. Because these companies reflect what we believe in. Our practice projects the way we focus our profession.

In my case, SOHO is aligned with my values, with my background, with my purpose. Every decision (location, business model, target...) is the result of exhaustive analysis. If I compare SOHO's planning to other practices, I can say that it is a project with greater maturity and authenticity. This is the result of guided reflection and planning.

Combining your passions in your company makes the project even more exciting. Architecture is something that has fascinated me since I was a child. I could say I'm a frustrated architect! Design awakens my most creative side. It had to be an important element in this project. SOHO dental® is located in an emblematic building designed by Rafael de la Hoz, an architect whom I deeply admire. From its glass walkways you can see the sea, another essential element that was part of the concept that shapes SOHO.

We create what we believe in:

- SOHO is comprehensive, holistic and minimally invasive dentistry.
- SOHO is excellence, through a management model that helps us measure, analyze and improve.
- SOHO is innovation, in the business model and in new technologies applied to diagnosis and treatment.

- SOHO is experience, in which we work on the five senses with our patient, team and collaborators.
- SOHO is design and passion for architecture, because the environment is important.
- SOHO is a healthy lifestyle, because it is our way of understanding health.
- SOHO is sustainability, because we respect the environment.
- SOHO is social responsibility, because we believe in a better world through the sum of small actions.
- SOHO is training, because we are passionate about teaching and learning (SOHO Academy®).
- SOHO is a way of understanding dentistry. SOHO is a philosophy.

SOHO is the result.

WATCH

Video:
*SOHO Dental, the result*

Your future is your present, i.e., every decision and every action you make will take you to the place you want to be.

You and only you design your reality.

M_CONCEPT is not only a management tool; it is a guide that invites you to reflect and that orients you on the path to follow to achieve your own objectives.

You have a great opportunity to do what really makes you happy and to add value through your talent.

The world needs people like you to evolve.

The possibility of realizing a dream is what makes life interesting.

*This book is dedicated to you, to those professionals for whom dentistry is your ikigai.*

## Special mention

I couldn't finish this book without making a special mention of my mentor, Brian Swann.

Many professionals have been involved in this *connecting the dots* theory, who have guided me, from whom I have learned and whom I deeply admire.

There are people who mark your career, not only professionally, but personally, making you see the world from another perspective. For me, Brian Swann is one of these.

Thank you for all you have contributed to dentistry.

Thank you for your dedication to teaching, to the profession and to the people around you.

To the entire team of professionals who are part of the Harvard School of Dental Medicine (HSDM) and Harvard Business School (HBS), from whom I have learned so much, thank you.

WATCH

Video
Dean B. Donoff

## Learn more about M_CONCEPT

M_CONCEPT is a model developed by MBA dental®.

MBA dental® is the first MBA oriented towards dentists with this unique model, based on differentiation through excellence and innovation.

The teaching methodology has an eminently practical approach, is 100% adapted to dental practices and provides results after it is implemented.

V I S I T

MBA dental® is presented in two modalities: one is 100% online and one is semi-distance learning. You can take the European or Latin American edition (visit our website to see the venues and the complete program).

## Keep it simple

Lean dental: digitize and simplify management.

This management model would be complex without a system that allows us to analyze, in a simple way, all the data we are going to work with in our dental practice.

For this purpose, we have developed a software which integrates all information through a digital flow, from strategy to excellence (quality measurement). This way, we will not only optimize all processes, but also introduce our patient into the digital experience.

What does this program bring us?

- Integration of the M_CONCEPT model: modules that form part of each area.
- Dashboard: a comprehensive module that allows us to keep track of everything that happens in our dental practice at all times.
- Automation of processes: such as check in, check out, online appointments, satisfaction measurement, automated communication delivery (SMS, emailing, appointment reminders to our patients…).

V I S I T

## Dental Lifestyle®: management as you've never heard it before

Can you imagine learning management wherever and however you want with leaders in dentistry (Christian Coachman, Iván Malagón, Hugo Madeira…) and the teaching team at MBA dental®?

Dental Lifestyle® is a 100% online program that introduces you to management, based on the microlearning methodology (learning in doses). You can dedicate 15 minutes a day to it.

The contents are made up of interactive videos with theoretical content, an *e-book*, interviews, a forum and an audiovisual library. When the student joins DL, they have unlimited access to the platform forever.

VISIT

## Stay in touch with us

This is only the beginning. We want to get to know you. If you want to share your experience, meet our team or be part of our MBA dental® family, please contact us at:

Web: https://mbadental.proE-mail: info@mbadental.pro

Instagram:

@m_conceptthebook

@mba_dental.pro

@dentallifestyle.es

@laurasanmartin

# Bibliography


1. Kaufman, J. *The personal MBA: Master the art of business.* Nueva York: Portfolio; 2012.
2. Porter, M.E. *Estrategia competitiva: técnicas para el análisis de los sectores industriales y de la competencia.* México D. F: Cecsa; 2000.
3. Kawasaki, G. *The art of the start.* Múnich: Vahlen; 2014.
4. Harvard Business Review. *HBR guide to setting your strategy.* Boston: Harvard Business Review Press; 2020.
5. Osterwalder, A. y Pigneur, Y. *Generación de modelos de negocio. Un manual para visionarios, revolucionarios y retadores.* Barcelona: Ediciones Deusto; 2011.
6. Mullins, J. *The new business road test: What entrepreneurs and executives should do before writing a business plan.* 3.ª ed. Nueva Jersey: FT Press; 2010.
7. Osterwalder, A., Pigneur, Y. y Smith, A. *La empresa invencible.* Barcelona: Urano; 2020.
8. Blank, S. y Dorf, B. *El manual del emprendedor.* Barcelona: Gestión 2000; 2016.
9. Edge, J. *Agile: Una guía esencial sobre la gestión de proyectos Agile, el proceso Kanban y el Lean Thinking + Una guía completa sobre Scrum.* Gloucester: Bravex Publications; 2020.
10. Harvard Business School Press. *Making Smart Decisions.* Boston: Harvard Business Review Press; 2006.
11. Gothelf, J. *Lean UX: Applying lean principles to improve user experience.* Sebastopol (California): O'Reilly Media; 2013.
12. Porter, M.E. *Ventaja competitiva - Creación y sostenimiento de un desempeño superior.* México: Compañía Editorial Continental; 1998.
13. McCarthy, R. *El método Agile.* Autoedición; 2020.
14. Joyal, F. *Everything is marketing. The Ultimate Strategy for Dental Practice Growth. 5.ª ed. Utah: Vevante;* 2014.
15. Ochoa de Aspuru, A. *Actitud salmón.* Amazon; 2020.
16. Godin, S. *Esto es marketing.* Madrid: Alienta Editorial; 2019.
17. Godin, S. *La vaca púrpura.* Barcelona: Gestión 2000; 2019.
18. Lindstrom, M. *Buyology: Truth and lies about why we buy.* Nueva York: Bantam Doubleday Dell; 2010.
19. Few, S. *Show me the numbers: Designing tables and graphs to enlighten.* Oakland: Analytics Press; 2012.
20. Kenny, G. What are your KPIs really measuring? *Harvard Business Review* [Internet], 2020 [consultado el 28 de mayo de 2021]. Disponible en: https://hbr.org/2020/09/what-are-your-kpis-really-measuring
21. Hobbs, O.H. *Accounting made simple: Accounting explained in 100 pages or less.* Createspace; 2015.
22. Altman, H. *Lean Analytics: Enfócate en datos que realmente importen para tu empresa.* Autoedición; 2018.
23. Koomey, J.G. *Turning numbers into knowledge.* Terre Haute: Wish Publishing; 2003.
24. Kiyosaki, R.T. *Padre rico padre pobre para jóvenes.* Barcelona: Debolsillo; 2020.
25. Koch, R. *El principio 80/20: el secreto de lograr más con menos.* Barcelona: Ediciones Paidós Ibérica; 2009.
26. Sinek, S. *Start with Why.* Nueva York: Portfolio; 2013.
27. Covey, S.R. *Los 7 hábitos de la gente altamente efectiva.* Barcelona: Planeta; 2012.
28. Andersen, E. *Growing great employees: Turning ordinary people into extraordinary performers.* Nueva York: Portfolio; 2008.

29. CIALDINI, R. *Pre-Suasion / Per-Suation*. Estados Unidos: Conecta; 2017.
30. CHAN, K.W. y MAUBORGNE, R.A. *Blue ocean strategy: How to create uncontested market space and make the competition irrelevant*. Boston: Harvard Business Review Press; 2005.
31. PETERS, T. *The Circle of Innovation: You Can't Shrink Your Way to Greatness*. Nueva York: Vintage Books; 2010.
32. BLANK, S. *The four steps to the epiphany: Successful strategies for products that win*. Nashville: John Wiley & Sons; 2020.
33. RIES, E. *El método Lean Startup*. Barcelona: Deusto; 2018.
34. DRUCKER, P.F. *La innovación y el empresario innovador*. Barcelona: Edhasa; 1997.
35. BERKUN, S. *The myths of innovation*. 1.ª ed. Sebastopol (California): O'Reilly Media; 2010.
36. HARVARD BUSINESS REVIEW. *HBR guide to thinking strategically (HBR guide series)*. Boston: Harvard Business Review Press; 2019.
37. COLLINS, J. *Good to Great*. Barcelona: Editorial Reverté; 2021.
38. MAURYA, A. *Running Lean*. Sebastopol (California): O'Reilly Media; 2014.
39. PETERS, T.J. y WATERMAN, R.H. *En busca de la excelencia*. Nashville: Harper Collins; 2017.
40. GOLDRATT, E.M. y COX, J. *La meta: un proceso de mejora continua*. 3.ª ed. Madrid: Diaz de Santos; 2005.
41. ROVIRA CELMA, A. *La buena suerte*. Barcelona: Urano; 2016.
42. WOOLLEY K. y FISHBACH, A. What separates goals we achieve from goals we don't. *Harvard Business Review* [Internet], 2017 [consultado el 31 de mayo de 2021]. Disponible en: https://hbr.org/2017/04/what-separates-goals-we-achieve-from-goals-we-dont
43. CLEAR, J. *Atomic habits: An easy & proven way to build good habits & break bad ones*. Nueva York: Avery Publishing Group; 2018.
44. SCOTT, A. *Loserthink*. Barcelona: Urano; 2020.
45. CUDDY, A. *Presence: Bringing your boldest self to your biggest challenges*. Nueva York: Back Bay Books; 2018.
46. MEYER, C. y SCHWAGER A. Comprendiendo la experiencia del cliente. *Harvard Business Review*, 2007; 85(2):89-99.
47. FEINSTEIN, A. Why you should be writing down your goals. *Forbes Magazine* [Internet], 2014 [consultado el 31 de mayo de 2021]. Disponible en: https://www.forbes.com/sites/ellevate/2014/04/08/why-you-should-be-writing-down-your-goals/
48. HARVARD BUSINESS ESSENTIALS. *Comunicación empresarial: Una guía para directivos ocupados*. Madrid: Deusto; 2007.
49. BUCKHOLTZ, J.W., TREADWAY, M.T., COWAN, R.L., *et al*. Dopaminergic Network Differences in Human Impulsivity. *Science*, 2010; 329(5991):532.
50. ACHOR, S. *The happiness advantage: The seven principles of positive psychology that fuel success and performance at work*. Nueva York: Random House; 2010.
51. JOLLEY, W. *Actitud de Excelencia!* Florida: Tdee; 2010.

# Collaborators

Forewords:

Brian Swann. Assistant Professor at Harvard School of Dental Medicine (HSDM).

Iván Malagón. Orthodontics expert, opinion leader and international speaker.

Dr. Arturo Arciniega. Expert in Cosmetic Dentistry.

Dr. Ashiana Jivraj. Dentist at the HSDM and at the MBA Harvard Business School (HBS).

Carlo Gallucci Calabrese. Professor at the Department of Marketing at Esade and Vice-rector for International Relations and Students at Ramon Llull University.

Dean B. Donoff. Professor Emeritus and Dean of Harvard School of Dental Medicine (HSDM).

Fernando Botella. Business trainer and writer.

Francesco Magani. Expert in Aesthetic Dentistry.

Fred Joyal. Dental Marketing Expert and author of the book *Everything is marketing*.

Ignacio Pedrinaci. Dentist, Periodontics EFP Board and ITI fellow at the HSDM.

Dr. Kyle Stanley. Dentist, Chief Clinical Officer at Pearl AI and international speaker.

Dr. Lewis Chen. Dentist, Co-founder of Beam Street and lecturer.

# Acronyms and abbreviations

AMA: American Marketing Association
KMI: Knowledge-method-implementation
WC: Working capital
BM: Business model
NPS: Net Promoter Score
OKR: Objectives and Key Results
DCP: Dental care process
PDP: Pre-during-post
MP: Marketing plan
BP: Business plan
PJ: Patient journey
PJM: Patient Journey Map
PPS: People-processes-structure
SASO: Systematization, analysis, stabilization-standardization and optimization
TQM: Total Quality Management
VUCA: Volatility, uncertainty, complexity and ambiguity